366 SIMPLE AND DELICIOUS WAYS TO STAY HEALTHY, VIGOROUS, AND YOUNG

Start with the Salmon-stuffed Cherry Tomatoes appetizer before moving on to the Fillet of Sole Roll-ups with Carrot Filling. Complement these with a Sautéed Radicchio Salad and top it all off with a big helping of Easiest Peaches Melba. In addition to the creative dishes and healthful tips, you'll find:

- A full explanation of the role each antioxidant plays in maintaining good health
- How phytochemicals work with antioxidants to kill harmful free radicals in the body
- Innovative ideas for vegetable and fruit side dishes, breads and muffins, grains and salads
- Menus for complete meals
- A detailed nutritional analysis of calories, fat grams, percentage of calories from fat, protein, fiber, calcium, sodium, and cholesterol for each recipe

Make every day of the year a healthy adventure with . . .

Antioxidant Power

Dolores Riccio is the author of *Superfoods, Superfoods for Women, 366 Delicious Ways to Cook Pasta with Vegetables,* and *Superfoods for Life.* She lives in Warwick, Rhode Island.

Also by Dolores Riccio

Superfoods

Superfoods for Women

Superfoods for Life

366 Delicious Ways to Cook Pasta with Vegetables

Antioxidant Power

366 DELICIOUS RECIPES FOR GREAT HEALTH AND LONG LIFE

DOLORES RICCIO

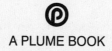

A PLUME BOOK

Ed Blonz, Ph.D., is a nationally syndicated columnist and author of *Your Personal Nutritionist* series (Signet, 1996). He is president of Nutrition Resource. Nutrition analysis was supplied using the Nutritionist IV™ software.

PLUME
Published by the Penguin Group
Penguin Putnam Inc., 375 Hudson Street, New York, New York 10014, U.S.A.
Penguin Books Ltd, 27 Wrights Lane, London W8 5TZ, England
Penguin Books Australia Ltd, Ringwood, Victoria, Australia
Penguin Books Canada Ltd, 10 Alcorn Avenue, Toronto, Ontario, Canada M4V 3B2
Penguin Books (N.Z.) Ltd, 182–190 Wairau Road, Auckland 10, New Zealand

Penguin Books Ltd, Registered Offices: Harmondsworth, Middlesex, England

First published by Plume, a member of Penguin Putnam Inc.

First Printing, February, 1999

1 3 5 7 9 10 8 6 4 2

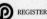 REGISTERED TRADEMARK—MARCA REGISTRADA

LIBRARY OF CONGRESS CATALOGING-IN-PUBLICATION DATA:
Riccio, Dolores, 1931–
Antioxidant power : 366 delicious recipes for great health and long life / Dolores Riccio.
p. cm.
Includes index.
ISBN 0-452-27728-0
1. Nutrition.   2. Antioxidants.   I. Title.
RA784.R4978   1999
613.2'6—dc21   98-38178
CIP

Printed in the United States of America
Set in Garamond Light and Avenir

BOOKS ARE AVAILABLE AT QUANTITY DISCOUNTS WHEN USED TO PROMOTE PRODUCTS OR SERVICES. FOR INFORMATION PLEASE WRITE TO PREMIUM MARKETING DIVISION, PENGUIN PUTNAM INC., 375 HUDSON STREET, NEW YORK, NEW YORK 10014.

To Rick whose faith and love always sustain me.

ACKNOWLEDGMENTS

My warmest thanks
to my editor, Jennifer Moore, for her thoughtful stewardship
of this cookbook,
to my super agent, Blanche Schlessinger, for her wisdom,
enthusiasm, and encouragement,
to my friend, Joan Bingham, for her expert help in
testing and commenting,
and to all those people who make cooking, for me, an extension of love,
friends and family who enjoy the pleasure of sharing earth's
bounty together.

Contents

Introduction: Antioxidants to the Rescue!

ANTIOXIDANTS DEFEND US AGAINST AGE

*A*ntioxidants* may be defined as any substance that protects tissue against oxidative damage. Even though oxygen is our primary fuel and we need a constant supply to live, when we use this fuel to generate energy, waste products are spewed off that are damaging. Just as an old car gets rusty or a piece of apple left out on a dish turns brown, these waste products cause us to degenerate faster—that is, to show the signs of age and to be more vulnerable to disease.

ANTIOXIDANT NUTRIENTS ARE OLD FRIENDS

Antioxidant nutrients are just another name for a group of familiar vitamins and minerals that have been around for decades. We learned about them first in a negative way, that if we didn't have enough of one or another, a disease of deficiency would surely result. So the U.S. government developed standards, Recommended Daily Allowances or RDAs for each of these vitamins and minerals.

More recently, however, nutritional and medical researchers have discovered that antioxidants play a much more vital role in health and well-being than was previously thought possible for mere nutrients. (Some major studies addressing this and other nutritional issues include the Nurses' Health Study begun in 1976, which involved over 87,000 female nurses for eight years, and the Health Professionals Study, which followed nearly 40,000 male subjects—doctors, dentists, and other medical personnel—over a four-year period.) A preponderance of current research concludes that antioxidants can help prevent the major diseases responsible for thousands of deaths every year and many other illnesses caused or encouraged by oxidative damage.

Antioxidant nutrients are being credited with averting or delaying heart disease, cancer, cataracts, neurological disease, and some of the effects of aging. It's entirely possible that many people could be lowering their risk of disease by increasing their intake of antioxidant foods. Antioxidants have therefore become the stars of current nutritional research.

UNCONTROLLED FREE RADICALS ARE THE CULPRITS

Oxidative damage is caused by substances called *free radicals*—incomplete, highly unstable oxygen atoms that cause harm to our cells and tissues. A free radical carries an unmated electron that wants urgently to pair up with another. This need propels an uncontrolled free radical into taking an electron from a neighboring molecule. The looting of healthy molecules leads to the faulty metabolism of proteins, DNA, and enzymes, comparable to rust and spoilage in items left to the ravages of open air. The injury done by free radicals is implicated in over fifty killer diseases.

Although our bodies have a built-in system for mopping up free radicals, this response may be swamped by an overload of free radicals or may lose its effectiveness with age. Uncontrolled free radicals bombard our cells constantly from within and without. Inside the body they are spewed out as a product of every normal biological process, since all cells require oxygen to generate energy, with its downside, oxidative damage. Outside the body, too, are many invisible potential enemies. Free radicals invade us from sources such as pollution, radiation, cigarette smoke, organic solvents, and herbicides. They assault us, too, in our recovery from traumatic wounds or burns, unusual exercise, or emotional stress. Once loose in the body, uncontrolled free radicals bond indiscriminately to whatever is handy, including vital DNA molecules, causing chain reactions that lead to cancerous mutations, impaired energy output, compromised immunity, and premature aging. They even may cause neurological degeneration such as Parkinson's and Alzheimer's diseases.

Yet our bodies can't get along without *controlled free radicals*, the ones that are necessary to sustain life. White blood cells in the immune system, for instance, use free radicals to bond to invading bacteria and viruses, the better to destroy them. Free radicals are also a necessary part of many metabolic processes. But whenever free radicals are not given an occupation, they run wild in the system and are generally bad news.

THE ANTIOXIDANT TEAM NEUTRALIZES FREE RADICALS

Although new antioxidant properties in food chemicals are constantly being discovered, *the basic antioxidant team is made up of three vitamins and two minerals*. They are *provitamin A* (carotene), *vitamin C*, *vitamin E*, and the minerals *selenium* and *zinc*. This group comprises the first food defense in aiding the body to fight the effects of free radicals. Antioxidants are able to sponge up hosts of free radicals and neutralize them before they cause the malfunctions that lead to the diseases and disorders characteristic of aging.

Antioxidant foods give you a supercharged immunity, and much more. They also enhance appearance by protecting hair, skin, teeth, gums, and nails. They postpone wrinkles and may even protect against skin injury from too much sun exposure. And they safeguard the reproductive systems of both men and women. What you eat is a most important contribution to your immune system.

ANTIOXIDANT FOODS ARE MORE POTENT THAN ANTIOXIDANT SUPPLEMENTS

The finest food sources of antioxidant vitamins and minerals—many of them fruits and vegetables—also contain numerous antioxidant *phytochemicals*. These plant chemicals, developed by plants to protect them from extreme weather conditions and natural predators, have been found to defend humans as well, and they are currently being studied by nutrition scientists for their far-reaching protective qualities. The presence of these additional compounds may explain why antioxidant foods do a better job of sponging up free radicals than supplements.

For example, in a recent study at the U.S. Department of Agriculture, researchers found that ¾ of a cup of kale, which contains only 40 mg of vitamin C and 10 IU of vitamin E, inactivated as many free radicals as supplements containing 500 mg of vitamin C and over 800 IU of vitamin E. This is an outstanding success of food over isolated vitamins.

Other winners (besides kale) in this competition were apples, bananas, beets, blueberries, broccoli, brussels sprouts, cabbage, carrots, cauliflower, corn, eggplant, grapes, grapefruit (pink), green beans, lettuce (leafy), onions, oranges, potatoes, pears, peppers (red bell), plums, spinach, strawberries, and tomatoes.

This was a limited test tube study, which means two things: that the action of these foods in the body might be different than in the test tube and that other foods may have made the list if they had been studied. Still, it's a pretty impressive vote of confidence for foods over pills.

All the antioxidant nutrients can be abundantly found in foods *except vitamin E*. In order to obtain a good supply of vitamin E, you need to be vigilant and thoughtful in menu planning, and religious about substituting vitamin E–rich vegetable oils for other kinds of fats. If this proves to be a difficult course, a vitamin E supplement or a one-a-day containing vitamin E might prove to be good insurance. But food should always be the first choice.

Choosing antioxidant foods is good for us in tangential ways as well. They provide a great deal of fiber but very little saturated fat. Even the vegetable oils that supply vitamin E are largely unsaturated. One of the most important, olive oil, is monounsaturated, a kind of oil that is actually credited with improving the cholesterol picture.

GOOD TASTING AS WELL AS GOOD FOR YOU

Happily, the important antioxidant foods are delicious as well as nutritious. A diet high in antioxidants is a diet high in fiber and low in saturated fat. These foods are readily available and easy to prepare in quick, tasty dishes, such as are described throughout this cookbook. From earthy to elegant, dishes rich in antioxidants can be equally at home in entertaining guests as well as at the family dinner table.

Vitamin A and the Carotenoids

Provitamin A (the vegetable form of vitamin A) is best known as *beta-carotene*, although other carotenoids are also important. Think of deep yellow, orange, and dark green foods when you think of beta-carotene.

Think of red foods like tomatoes, red bell peppers, and watermelon for *lycopene*, a carotenoid cousin. These two—beta-carotene and lycopene—are credited with lessening the risk of oral, esophageal, reproductive, lung, colon, stomach, cervix, and prostate cancers. (Some of the strongest relationships are between beta-carotene and lung cancer, vitamin C and stomach cancer, vitamin E and heart disease.)

Think of dark green foods like broccoli and mustard greens for *lutein* and *zeaxanthin*, other carotenoid relatives responsible for keeping the eyes healthy throughout life.

The best food choices for provitamin A are apricots, carrots, dark greens, melons, mangoes, nectarines, papayas, peaches, potatoes (sweet), pumpkin, red bell peppers and red chilies, winter squash, and tomatoes.

Vitamin C

An immune-system enhancer and wound healer, vitamin C has been shown to be especially effective as a cancer fighter. Research evidence indicates that vitamins C and E together are important in preventing cardiovascular disease. A good supply of these complementary nutrients actually decreases a dangerous thickening of carotid artery walls, the main blood vessels supplying the brain. A low intake of vitamin C can also be related to infertility.

Vitamin C is a skin vitamin, too, encouraging the production of collagen, a substance that repairs skin. This important vitamin also wards off asthma and protects against gum disease.

The best food choices for vitamin C are berries, broccoli, brussels sprouts, cabbage, citrus fruits, kale, kiwifruit, melons, pineapple, parsley, peas, potatoes, and tomatoes. Apples, beets, pears, and plums contain some vitamin C as well.

Vitamin E

Vitamin E helps to block the cell damage that leads to aging and cancer. It protects against heart attacks and strokes by reducing the harmful effects of LDL cholesterol and preventing blood clots. It is necessary for normal cell respiration, membrane protection, and kidney, genital, and nervous system function.

Unlike other antioxidants, which are plentiful in many foods, sources of vitamin E are few and the quantities limited. Some of the best vitamin E foods are high in fat (but not saturated fat) and calories. The way to combat this problem is to eat less fat overall but choose vitamin E oils when you use fats for cooking or in salads. The recipes in this book often use olive oil, an excellent source of vitamin E. As a monounsaturated fat, olive oil is beneficial in controlling cholesterol.

The best food choices for vitamin E are asparagus, avocados, brussels sprouts, dark greens, nuts and seeds, oils, mangoes, tomatoes, seafood, and whole grains.

Selenium

This essential mineral is a dynamic team player, enhancing many benefits of vitamin E. Selenium helps to preserve elasticity as we grow older. There is good evidence that selenium boosts the immune system in general. More specifically, in a recent controlled study of the effects of selenium on human subjects, it reduced the risk of prostate, colon, and lung cancer from 40 to 63 percent. The subjects of this study lived in an area where the selenium content of soil (and therefore of locally grown produce) is very low, which may have made the findings more dramatic. Nevertheless, selenium's power as a disease fighter seems indisputable.

Beware of selenium supplements, however; this mineral can be toxic at high levels. The greatest food source of selenium—other than seafood—is Brazil nuts. It would not be a good idea, for instance, to combine a selenium supplement with a helping of Brazil nuts.

The best food choices for selenium are asparagus, nuts, mushrooms, seafood and shellfish, seeds, wheat germ, and whole grains.

Zinc

Sometimes called the unsung antioxidant, zinc's role as an antioxidant mineral is to sponge up some of the most common and abundant free radicals. Zinc is also essential for general healing, and it fortifies the immune system. A deficiency in zinc lessens the sense of taste. This mineral is also an important protector of male reproductive ability.

The best food choices for zinc are dairy products, legumes, nuts, barley, brown rice, seeds, shellfish, turkey, wheat germ, and whole grains.

The Fabulous Antioxidant Foods

Apples
Apricots
Avocados
Bananas
Berries
Citrus fruits
Grapes
Kiwifruit
Mangoes
Melons

Nectarines
Papayas
Peaches
Pears
Plums

Barley
Cornmeal, whole grain
Nuts and seeds
Quinoa
Rice, brown
Wheat germ and whole grains

Dairy products
Seafood
Shellfish, especially oysters
Poultry, especially turkey

Asparagus
Beans, green and dried, lentils
Beets
Broccoli
Brussels sprouts
Cabbage
Carrots
Cauliflower
Corn
Eggplant
Greens and lettuce, dark leafy
Mushrooms
Onions
Peas, green and dried
Peppers and hot chilies
Potatoes, white and sweet
Pumpkin
Spinach
Squash, winter
Tomatoes

Oils: soybean, sesame, sunflower, peanut, flaxseed, olive

If we make these fabulous antioxidant foods a major part of our daily meals, we'll be giving ourselves an easy, readily available, effective means of staying healthy and vigorous throughout life. The recipes in this book focus on the goal of enriching us with antioxidant foods. Enjoy them and share them with the knowledge that they are both good tasting and good for you.

A Few Useful Basics

Here is a collection of recipes for basic ingredients such as chicken and vegetable stocks, tomato sauce, cooked beans, and salad dressings that are often used in making the recipes in this book. Although most of these products have their counterparts in store-bought items, if you have the time and inclination, homemade always tastes best.

Chicken Stock with a Bonus

---■---

The "bonus" is the lovely cooked chicken, which can be used for so many quick, satisfying dishes.

3 pounds split chicken breasts, with bones, skinned (4 pieces)
1 tablespoon olive oil
1 large onion, chopped
½ cup chopped shallots or scallions
2 celery stalks with leaves, chopped
1 teaspoon chopped fresh thyme, rosemary, and tarragon (choose any two or all three)

Several sprigs fresh parsley or cilantro, chopped
¼ cup no-salt or low-sodium tomato puree
½ teaspoon salt
2 large carrots, each cut into 2 pieces
⅛ to ¼ teaspoon pepper, to taste

Wash the chicken in salted cold water; rinse and drain.

In a large pot, heat the oil, add the onion, shallots, and celery, and "sweat" the vegetables over very low heat until lightly colored, about 10 minutes. Add the chopped herbs (except parsley) during the last minute. Remove the vegetables and lightly brown the chicken pieces.

Return the vegetables to the pot. Add 8½ cups water, the parsley, tomato puree, and salt. Cover and simmer the broth for 40 minutes. Add the carrots and pepper; continue cooking for 10 to 15 minutes. Strain the stock. Reserve the chicken and carrots for another use.

Kilocalories 40Kc • Protein 3 gm • Fat 1 gm • Percent of calories from fat 20% • Cholesterol 2 mg • Dietary fiber 0 gm • Sodium 42 mg • Calcium 0 mg

Vegetable-Tomato Stock

MAKES 8 CUPS

This all-purpose meatless soup stock will add flavor to vegetarian dishes.

2 tablespoons olive oil
1 onion, chopped
1 bunch scallions with tops, chopped
3 garlic cloves, finely chopped
4 celery stalks with leaves, chopped
2 large carrots, chopped
1 green bell pepper, seeded and chopped
6 outside leaves romaine lettuce or escarole

1 (1-pound) can no-salt or low-sodium chopped tomatoes with juice
1 tablespoon chopped fresh basil
Several sprigs of fresh parsley, chopped
½ teaspoon salt
⅛ to ¼ teaspoon pepper

Heat the oil in a large pot. Add the vegetables, except tomatoes, and "sweat" them over very low heat until they are lightly colored, 15 to 20 minutes. Add 8 cups of water, tomatoes, herbs, and salt. Simmer covered for 1 hour. Stir in the pepper. Strain before using, pressing on the solids to extract as much liquid as possible.

Kilocalories 40 Kc • Protein 1 gm • Fat 1 gm • Percent of calories from fat 10% • Cholesterol 0 mg • Dietary fiber 0 gm • Sodium 42 mg • Calcium 0 mg

A FEW USEFUL BASICS

11

Polenta Pronto

■

MAKES 3½ CUPS, 4 SERVINGS

Here's a polenta recipe that doesn't require a half hour of stirring at the stove—just some brisk whisking and a large double boiler.

1 cup polenta (coarsely ground cornmeal, preferably whole grain)

2 cups chicken or vegetable stock (pages 10, 11) or low-sodium canned broth

½ cup freshly grated Parmesan cheese (loosely packed)

¼ teaspoon white pepper

In a 4-cup measuring pitcher, blend the polenta with 2 cups of cold water. Pour the stock into the top of a double boiler. Bring it to a boil over direct heat. Gradually add the polenta mixture, stirring with a whisk to prevent clumping. Lower the heat and keep stirring until the polenta thickens, about 3 minutes. (Keep the simmer low enough to prevent splattering of hot polenta.)

Meanwhile, bring 2 inches of water to a boil in the bottom of the double boiler. Place the top of the double boiler with the polenta over the simmering water. Cook with cover slightly ajar for 45 minutes. Briskly whisk every 15 minutes to smooth any lumps.

Remove the polenta from the heat. Whisk in the cheese and pepper. Serve hot, topped with any of a variety of sauces. Or chill in an 11 × 7-inch pan, and when firm, cut into squares. Warm or fry the squares when ready to add the topping.

Kilocalories 192 Kc • Protein 9 gm • Fat 4 gm • Percent of calories from fat 19% • Cholesterol 9 mg • Dietary fiber 3 gm • Sodium 212 mg • Calcium 142 mg

Basil Pesto

MAKES ABOUT 2 CUPS, 16 SERVINGS

This pesto has plenty of vitamin E–rich pine nuts, as well as vitamins A and C in the basil.

1 cup pine nuts
2 garlic cloves, halved
3 to 4 cups fresh basil leaves, spun very dry, well packed (see Note)
½ teaspoon salt

¼ teaspoon freshly ground black pepper
About ½ cup olive oil
½ cup freshly grated Parmesan cheese (optional)

In a small unoiled skillet, toast the pine nuts over very low heat until they just begin to change color, about two minutes. Immediately transfer them to a dish, since they may overbrown if left in the hot pan.

In a food processor with the motor running, toss the garlic down the feed tube to mince it. Add the basil, pine nuts, salt, and pepper. Process until very finely chopped.

With the motor running, add the oil in a thin stream until the mixture is thick but not runny. Stop the motor once or twice to scrape the bottom and sides of the workbowl with a rubber spatula.

Stir in the cheese, if using. Transfer the pesto to a jar and pour a thin layer of oil on top to preserve the color. Cover and refrigerate until needed.

The pesto will keep for a week to 10 days—or it may be frozen for longer storage. A handy way of freezing this useful basic is to spray ice-cube trays with nonstick cooking spray, fill them with the pesto, and when they are solidly frozen, remove them to a plastic container.

NOTE: While basil turns dark when processed, parsley does not. For a brighter green color in the finished pesto, substitute 1 cup fresh flat-leaf parsley leaves for 1 cup basil in the preceding recipe.

Kilocalories 119 Kc • Protein 3 gm • Fat 12 gm • Percent of calories from fat 85% • Cholesterol 0 mg • Dietary fiber 1 gm • Sodium 73 mg • Calcium 16 mg

A FEW USEFUL BASICS

PARSLEY PESTO: Follow the preceding recipe, using fresh flat-leaf parsley instead of basil. Omit the cheese.

MAKES ABOUT 1 1/2 CUPS, 12 SERVINGS

Kilocalories 161 Kc • Protein 4 gm • Fat 16 gm • Percent of calories from fat 84% • Cholesterol 0 mg • Dietary fiber 1 gm • Sodium 106 mg • Calcium 25 mg

Tomato Sauce, Light and Spicy

■

MAKES 6 TO 7 CUPS,
ENOUGH TO SAUCE 2 POUNDS OF PASTA

Enriched with basil pesto, this sauce imparts the fresh taste of summer. If you make a batch of fresh pesto for this purpose, you can freeze the extra in an ice-cube tray.

1/3 cup olive oil
1 dry hot red chili
1 green bell pepper, seeded and diced
2 garlic cloves, minced
1/4 cup no-salt or low-sodium tomato paste
2 (28-ounce) cans imported Italian plum tomatoes in juice, undrained

1/2 teaspoon salt
1/2 teaspoon freshly ground black pepper
1 1/2 tablespoons (1 heaping) basil pesto (page 13, or from a jar), or 1 tablespoon minced fresh basil plus 1 tablespoon grated Parmesan cheese
1/4 cup chopped fresh flat-leaf parsley

Heat the oil in a large pot, and sauté the chili and bell pepper until the latter is softened, about 3 minutes. Add the garlic and cook for 1/2 minute. Add the tomato paste, and cook over very low heat, stirring very often, for 3 minutes. Add the plum tomatoes, salt, and pepper. Simmer the sauce, stirring occasionally, for 20 minutes. Remove the chili and break up the tomatoes with a potato masher. Return the chili to the sauce. Cook 30 to 40 minutes more, until it reaches a sauce consistency.

(If you used puree-packed instead of juice-packed tomatoes, this step will take less time.)

Stir in the basil pesto and parsley. Cook 3 to 5 minutes longer. Remove the chili before serving.

Kilocalories 175 Kc • Protein 2 gm • Fat 13 gm • Percent of calories from fat 68% • Cholesterol 0 mg • Dietary fiber 3 gm • Sodium 228 mg • Calcium 53 mg

TOMATO-MUSHROOM SAUCE: Clean and slice 10 ounces of small mushrooms—white, brown, or a mixture. In a large nonstick skillet, sauté the mushrooms over high heat in 2 tablespoons of olive oil, stirring often, until they release their juice and begin to brown. Salting the mushrooms helps this process. If you wish, you can also add a chopped shallot.

Follow the preceding recipe, adding the mushrooms with the tomatoes.

Kilocalories 217 Kc • Protein 3 gm • Fat 17 gm • Percent of calories from fat 69% • Cholesterol 0 mg • Dietary fiber 4 gm • Sodium 230 mg • Calcium 56 mg

Homemade Beans

■

MAKES 6 TO 8 CUPS—THE EQUIVALENT OF
3 (14- TO 16-OUNCE) CANS

Canned beans are a great time-saver for the busy cook, but homemade beans are tastier and less expensive. They take time but the actual preparation is easy.

The basic method for simmering dried beans is the same for all varieties. The timing varies, depending on the bean and the length of time it has been stored, not only in your pantry, but also in the store before purchase—so taste is the best test. Consult the chart that follows the basic recipe for timing and seasoning.

1 pound dried beans (2 to 2½ cups)	**1 garlic clove, minced (optional)**
1 tablespoon vegetable oil	**Herbs of your choice (page 17)**
1 onion, chopped	**½ teaspoon salt**
	Freshly ground black pepper

Spill the beans onto a tray, pick out any foreign material such as pebbles or twigs, and discard any shriveled beans. Rinse the beans thoroughly. Put the beans in a large pot, add 2 quarts of water, and put the beans in a cool place to soak overnight. The next day, drain and rinse the beans, discarding the soaking water.

If you want to cook more spontaneously, there is a faster method. Bring the beans and their soaking water to a boil, cook 2 minutes, remove them from the heat, and let them stand, covered, for 2 hours. As with the first method, drain and discard the soaking water.

Dry out the pot and heat the oil in it over low heat. Add the onion and garlic, if using; sauté them until they are sizzling and fragrant. Add the beans, 8 cups fresh cold water, and herbs of your choice. Bring to a very gentle simmer and cook, covered, until the beans are tender, stirring from time to time. Watch the water level and add more if needed.

Add the salt during the last few minutes of cooking time. Stir in pepper to taste. If there seems to be too much liquid, you can drain off some of it. Cooked beans freeze well and are convenient to have on hand.

Kilocalories 144 Kc • Protein 8 gm • Fat 2 gm • Percent of calories from fat 10% • Cholesterol 0 mg • Dietary fiber 9 gm • Sodium 106 mg • Calcium 52 mg

A Guide to Cooking and Seasoning Beans

Many herbs and spices are carminatives that reduce intestinal gas. Along with making a pot of beans more flavorful, herbs and spices also make them more digestible. Thyme, summer savory, dill, ginger, cilantro, fennel, and sage are all stomach soothers. A half tablespoon chopped fresh herbs or ½ teaspoon dried herbs is about right for a pot of beans.

Lentils and split peas do not appear on this chart. In general, they cook in less time and need no soaking. Recipes that use lentils and split peas give instructions for cooking them within the text.

Bean	Seasoning	Cooking Time After Soaking
Adzuki	Minced fresh ginger	1½ to 2 hours
Black beans	Orange peel slivers, thyme	1 to 1½ hours
Black-eyed peas	Summer savory or thyme	About 1 hour
Chickpeas (Garbanzos)	Fennel seeds or rosemary or fresh sage leaves Tomato paste (low-sodium)	1½ to 2 hours
Fava beans	Marjoram or rosemary or thyme	2 to 2½ hours
Kidney beans (Pink beans or red beans)	Dill or thyme or marjoram	1½ to 2 hours
White kidney beans (Cannellini)	Fennel seeds or rosemary	1½ to 2 hours
Lima beans	Dill, tomato paste	1 to 1½ hours
Navy beans (Pea beans)	Thyme	1½ to 2 hours
Pinto beans	Cilantro	1½ to 2 hours
Roman beans (Cranberry beans)	Oregano	1½ to 2 hours
Soybeans	Tomato paste (low-sodium), thyme	About 2 hours

Zesty Tomato Salsa

—■—

2 cups seeded chopped fresh plum tomatoes

1 seeded diced mild green (Anaheim) chili

1 to 2 seeded minced fresh jalapeño chilies (wear rubber gloves)

½ cup finely chopped scallions

1 garlic clove, crushed through a press

¼ cup fresh lime juice (2 limes)

2 tablespoons vegetable oil

2 tablespoons minced fresh cilantro or flat-leaf parsley

¼ teaspoon salt

¼ teaspoon freshly ground black pepper

Combine all the ingredients, stir well, and chill several hours or overnight to blend the flavors. Stir before serving.

Kilocalories 62 Kc • Protein 1 gm • Fat 5 gm • Percent of calories from fat 65% • Cholesterol 0 mg • Dietary fiber 1 gm • Sodium 105 mg • Calcium 15 mg

Boiled Shrimp

—■—

MAKES ABOUT 1 POUND, 3 TO 4 SERVINGS

1¼ pounds shrimp in shells

1 lemon, quartered and squeezed slightly

½ teaspoon salt

½ teaspoon whole peppercorns

Wash the shrimp well. (Wear rubber gloves.) Put the shrimp, lemon, salt, and peppercorns in a saucepan. Add water to cover. Bring the shrimp to a boil and simmer over very low heat for 3 minutes. Remove the pan from the heat and let the shrimp stand until they have all turned bright pink.

Drain the shrimp. When they're cool enough to handle, peel off the shells and remove the black vein that runs along the curved back of the shrimp.

Kilocalories 200 Kc • Protein 38 gm • Fat 3 gm • Percent of calories from fat 15% • Cholesterol 286 mg • Dietary fiber 0 gm • Sodium 281 mg • Calcium 98 mg

Garlic and Lemon Vinaigrette

■

MAKES 1 CUP, 8 SERVINGS

1 cup olive oil
Juice of 2 lemons (½ cup)
½ teaspoon dried oregano
2 garlic cloves, halved

¼ teaspoon salt
⅛ to ¼ teaspoon freshly ground
   black pepper

Combine all the ingredients in a jar or bottle and shake well. Allow the dressing to marinate at room temperature for a half hour or so before using.

If any dressing is left over, refrigerate it after discarding the garlic. Bring to room temperature and shake well before using.

Kilocalories 243 Kc • Protein 0 gm • Fat 27 gm • Percent of calories from fat 97% • Cholesterol 0 mg • Dietary fiber 0 gm • Sodium 73 mg • Calcium 4 mg

Herb Vinaigrette

■

⅔ cup olive oil
⅓ cup red wine vinegar
½ teaspoon salt
½ teaspoon freshly ground black
  pepper

1 tablespoon chopped chives
1 tablespoon chopped fresh
  marjoram or basil

Combine all the ingredients in a jar or bottle and shake well. Allow the dressing to marinate at room temperature for a half hour or so before using.

   If any dressing is left over, refrigerate it. Bring to room temperature and shake well before using.

Kilocalories 161 Kc • Protein 0 gm • Fat 18 gm • Percent of calories from fat 99% • Cholesterol 0 mg • Dietary fiber 0 gm • Sodium 145 mg • Calcium 5 mg

Dijon Vinaigrette

■

MAKES 1 CUP, 8 SERVINGS

3 tablespoons white wine
  vinegar
2 tablespoons Dijon mustard

About ¾ cup olive oil
¼ teaspoon freshly ground black
  pepper

In a blender, whisk together the vinegar and mustard. With the motor running, slowly pour the oil through the feed tube until the dressing is emulsified and thickened. Stir in the pepper. Refrigerate in a closed jar. Bring to room temperature and whisk before using.

Kilocalories 185 Kc • Protein 0 gm • Fat 21 gm • Percent of calories from fat 98% • Cholesterol 0 mg • Dietary fiber 0 gm • Sodium 22 mg • Calcium 6 mg

DIJON HONEY DRESSING: If you like a sweeter salad dressing, follow the preceding recipe and whisk in 1 tablespoon warmed honey with the pepper.

Kilocalories 193 Kc • Protein 0 gm • Fat 21 gm • Percent of calories from fat 94% • Cholesterol 0 mg • Dietary fiber 0 gm • Sodium 22 mg • Calcium 6 mg

Caesar Salad Dressing with Roasted Garlic

■

MAKES 1 CUP, 8 SERVINGS

Beside its use as a salad dressing, this savory mixture is also a delicious dip for raw vegetables.

1 whole bulb garlic
¼ cup white wine vinegar
¼ teaspoon freshly ground black pepper

4 anchovies, mashed
¾ cup extra-virgin olive oil

Preheat the oven to 375 degrees F.

Cut off the top of the garlic bulb and wrap the bulb in foil. Bake for 45 minutes, or until fragrant and soft when pressed. Cool the garlic enough to handle. Squeeze the garlic cloves out of their peels and mash them.

In a blender or food processor, blend together the garlic, vinegar, pepper, and anchovies. Gradually add the oil. Store in a widemouthed jar, refrigerated. Bring to room temperature before using. Whisk again just before measuring for salad.

Kilocalories 194 Kc • Protein 1 gm • Fat 20 gm • Percent of calories from fat 94% • Cholesterol 2 mg • Dietary fiber 0 gm • Sodium 75 mg • Calcium 16 mg

Appetizers and Snacks

The tempting spread of appetizers and snacks featured in this chapter are rich in antioxidant power and low in fat and salt, compared to the usual appetizer tray of smoked meats, hard cheeses, and salty crackers. Because these appetizers are "light," they stimulate rather than stifle the appetite for the main course.

Not necessarily for company, many of these little dishes make terrific treats to stash in the refrigerator for quick lunches or "snack attacks" at any time of day—especially any of the light cheese and vegetable platters. Some of them—such as Sicilian Eggplant Caponata, Antipasto Salad, Hummus, or Corn and Black Bean Salsa—can also double as great vegetarian sandwich fillings. And any of the bruschettas, of course, really are open-faced sandwiches, tasty on their own or as an accompaniment to a bowl of soup at lunchtime.

When you prepare several appetizers for a dinner party or buffet, the more choices you provide, the more people a recipe will serve because guests will eat less of each dish—in which case, the serving amounts given at the end of each recipe would be increased.

Bon appétit!

Garlic-and-Herb Yogurt Cheese with Veggies

MAKES 1¼ CUPS, 4 SERVINGS WITH THE VEGETABLES

You'll need to plan ahead for this tasty snack. The yogurt must be drained overnight to thicken to a cheese and then, when mixed with seasonings, will benefit from blending the flavors for several more hours.

2 cups nonfat plain yogurt
1 garlic clove, crushed through
 a press
½ teaspoon dried thyme
½ teaspoon dried basil
½ teaspoon dried dill
¼ teaspoon celery salt
Several dashes of black, white,
 and cayenne peppers

1 bunch radishes, washed and
 sliced
4 carrots, cut into sticks
1 large green bell pepper,
 seeded and cut into sticks
Whole wheat snack crackers

Set a paper coffee filter in a strainer that will hold 2 cups, spoon the yogurt into it, and set it over a bowl. Cover with plastic wrap. Allow the yogurt to drain overnight in the refrigerator.

The next day, remove the thickened yogurt to a bowl and discard the liquid. Add the garlic, thyme, basil, dill, celery salt, and peppers, blending well. Chill for several hours. When ready to serve, mound the yogurt on a plate, surround with radishes, carrots, and bell pepper, and place a basket of whole wheat crackers nearby.

Kilocalories 106 Kc • Protein 8 gm • Fat .26 gm • Percent of calories from fat 2% • Cholesterol 0 mg • Dietary fiber 3 gm • Sodium 114 mg • Calcium 258 mg

Curry and Onion Cheese with Shrimp and Vegetables

Make the yogurt cheese a day ahead of preparing this appetizer, a spicy dip that goes well with strong-flavored vegetables.

1 cup yogurt cheese
¼ cup mayonnaise
2 tablespoons chili sauce
1 teaspoon curry powder
2 tablespoons very finely
   chopped scallions

2 to 3 cups small raw broccoli
   and cauliflower florets (any
   ratio)
½ pound frozen cooked shelled
   and cleaned cocktail shrimp,
   thawed

Make the yogurt cheese as described in the preceding recipe.

   Blend the yogurt cheese with the mayonnaise, chili sauce, and curry powder. Stir in the scallions. Chill for several hours to blend the flavors. Surround the cheese with the vegetables and shrimp.

Kilocalories 238 Kc • Protein 19 gm • Fat 12 gm • Percent of calories from fat 45% • Cholesterol 121 mg • Dietary fiber 2 gm • Sodium 295 mg • Calcium 243 mg

APPETIZERS AND SNACKS

25

Crudités with Herb Aioli

MAKES ABOUT 1½ CUPS AIOLI,
8 SERVINGS WITH THE VEGETABLES

Here's a classic garlic mayonnaise that's lighter than traditional versions. Using an egg substitute not only lowers the cholesterol content, it also eliminates the health concerns connected with raw whole eggs.

For the aioli

About ¾ cup olive oil (or mixed with canola oil)
1 large garlic clove, minced
¼ cup prepared egg substitute
2 tablespoons white wine vinegar
¾ teaspoon salt
¼ teaspoon white pepper

1 tablespoon chopped fresh flat-leaf parsley
1 tablespoon chopped fresh basil
1 tablespoon chopped fresh marjoram
½ cup nonfat plain yogurt

For the crudités

2 green bell peppers, seeded and cut into strips
2 red bell peppers, seeded and cut into strips
1 bunch small radishes, trimmed and halved
2 cups small broccoli florets

3 large carrots, cut into sticks
3 small purple-topped turnips, sliced
1 fennel bulb, cored and sliced (do this at the last minute; fennel turns brown when exposed to the air)

In a small skillet, heat 1 tablespoon of the oil and sauté the garlic until it's sizzling. Remove from the heat and let stand while preparing the rest of the recipe.

In a blender or food processor, blend the egg substitute, vinegar, salt, and pepper. With the motor running, slowly pour the remaining oil down the feed tube until the mixture is as thick as desired. Briefly blend in the garlic; remove from the processor and chill. When ready to use, whisk in the fresh herbs and yogurt. Spoon into a bowl, surrounded by the vegetables.

Kilocalories 232 Kc • Protein 3 gm • Fat 21 gm • Percent of calories from fat 76% • Cholesterol 0 mg • Dietary fiber 3 gm • Sodium 280 mg • Calcium 73 mg

ANTIOXIDANT POWER

26

Guacamole

―――――――――――― ■ ――――――――――――

Serve this buttery, spicy blend with vegetable dippers and/or low-fat baked tortilla chips.

2 ripe avocados, peeled and halved, with pits removed

2 plum tomatoes, peeled, seeded, and chopped

2 scallions, chopped

1 fresh jalapeño chili, seeded and minced (wear rubber gloves)

Juice of 1 large lime (about 3 tablespoons)

½ teaspoon salt

¼ teaspoon freshly ground black pepper

½ teaspoon or more hot pepper sauce, such as Tabasco

2 tablespoons minced fresh cilantro

Vegetable dippers such as cucumber and radish slices, bell peppers, carrots, and celery sticks

Low-fat baked tortilla chips

In a food processor, blend the avocados, tomatoes, scallions, chili, lime juice, salt, pepper, and hot pepper sauce. Remove the mixture from the processor and stir in the cilantro. Taste to correct the seasoning. You may want more salt or hot pepper sauce. Serve with vegetable dippers and baked tortilla chips.

Kilocalories 110 Kc • Protein 2 gm • Fat 10 gm • Percent of calories from fat 75% • Cholesterol 0 mg • Dietary fiber 3 gm • Sodium 205 mg • Calcium 11 mg

APPETIZERS AND SNACKS

27

Hummus

Serve this spicy chickpea spread with sesame crackers or pita bread wedges. Leftovers make a tasty spread for toast to serve with soup.

2 tablespoons sesame seeds
4 tablespoons olive oil
1 yellow onion, chopped
2 garlic cloves, minced
2 cups homemade chickpeas (page 16) or 1 (15- to 16-ounce) can low-sodium chickpeas, drained and rinsed
2 tablespoons or more fresh lemon juice

½ teaspoon salt
¼ teaspoon freshly ground black pepper
Cayenne to taste
1 teaspoon chopped fresh thyme or ¼ teaspoon dried
1 teaspoon chopped fresh oregano or ¼ teaspoon dried
½ teaspoon ground cumin

In a small skillet, toast the sesame seeds until they turn golden, about 2 minutes over low heat, watching them carefully. Remove them from the pan promptly so that the remaining heat will not brown them.

In the same skillet, heat 2 tablespoons of the oil and sauté the onion and garlic until they are soft and fragrant but not brown, 3 to 5 minutes.

In a food processor, blend the chickpeas, lemon juice, salt, black pepper, cayenne, thyme, oregano, cumin, toasted sesame seeds, onion and garlic with their oil, plus the remaining 2 tablespoons of oil. Stop the motor to scrape down the sides once or twice. The mixture should be thick but creamy. Taste to correct the seasoning; you may want more salt or lemon juice.

Kilocalories 145 Kc • Protein 4 gm • Fat 9 gm • Percent of calories from fat 53% • Cholesterol 0 mg • Dietary fiber 4 gm • Sodium 151 mg • Calcium 50 mg

ANTIOXIDANT POWER

28

Pinto Bean Dip

■

This is great to snack on when watching TV brings on an attack of the "munchies."

1/4 medium red onion
1 garlic clove, peeled
2 cups homemade pinto beans
  (page 16) or 1 (14- to 16-ounce)
  can low-sodium pinto beans,
  drained and rinsed
1 large tomato, quartered
2 canned jalapeño chilies,
  seeded and chopped (wear
  rubber gloves)

2 teaspoons chili powder
1 teaspoon ground cumin
About 3 tablespoons olive oil
No-salt melba toasts, low-salt
  bagel chips, or low-fat baked
  tortilla chips as an
  accompaniment

In a food processor with the motor running, toss the onion and garlic down the feed tube to mince them. Add the beans, tomato, chilies, chili powder, and cumin. Gradually add enough oil to make a thick, smooth, creamy mixture. Stop the motor to scrape down the sides once or twice. Taste to correct the seasoning. You may want more chili powder or salt.

Chill to blend the flavors, but bring to room temperature before serving. Surround the dip with toasts or chips.

Kilocalories 148 Kc • Protein 5 gm • Fat 7 gm • Percent of calories from fat 42% • Cholesterol 0 mg • Dietary fiber 6 gm • Sodium 28 mg • Calcium 40 mg

APPETIZERS AND SNACKS

Baba Ghanouj with Roasted Garlic

MAKES 3 CUPS, 6 SERVINGS

This is an exotic and popular appetizer, made rich in vitamin E with sesame seed paste, available in natural food stores and many supermarkets.

2 large eggplants (1¼ to
  1½ pounds)
1 whole bulb garlic
½ cup tahini (see Note)
Juice of 2 to 3 lemons
1 cup nonfat plain yogurt
1 tablespoon chopped fresh
  parsley

1 tablespoon extra-virgin
  olive oil
Pita bread as an accompaniment
1 small red onion, chopped, as
  an accompaniment

Preheat the oven to 400 degrees F.

Prick the eggplants in several places with a fork. Cut off the top of the garlic bulb and wrap it in foil. Put the eggplants and garlic on a baking sheet and bake until they are quite soft when pressed with the back of a cooking fork, 45 to 55 minutes. If the garlic gets soft earlier, remove it. When both are cooked, allow them to cool until they can be handled.

Scrape the eggplant pulp from the peel into a large bowl. Squeeze the garlic pulp out of the skins and add that to the eggplant. Mash the two together with a potato masher. Blend the tahini and lemon juice. Taste to determine if you want more than the juice of 2 lemons. Fold in the yogurt. Sprinkle with the parsley and olive oil.

Serve the baba ghanouj at room temperature with wedges of pita bread and a small bowl of chopped red onion.

NOTE: Tahini is traditional, but you can substitute ¼ cup toasted sesame seeds plus 1 teaspoon sesame oil, both of which can be found in most supermarkets. The oil is generally shelved with Asian foods.

Kilocalories 237 Kc • Protein 10 gm • Fat 16 gm • Percent of calories from fat 57% • Cholesterol 0 mg • Dietary fiber 3 gm • Sodium 34 mg • Calcium 142 mg

Roasted Bell Pepper Relish

Use this sweet-and-sour pepper relish as an appetizer or to dress up any plain poultry or fish dish.

2 large red bell peppers
2 large green bell peppers
3 tablespoons olive oil
1 small onion, chopped
2 garlic cloves, minced

1 tablespoon sugar
¼ teaspoon salt
¼ cup red wine vinegar
Freshly ground black pepper

Preheat the broiler. Put the bell peppers on a baking sheet and broil them about 6 inches from the heat source until all sides are partly charred, 2 to 3 minutes per side, and the peppers are tender. Put them into a covered casserole or pan to allow the steam to loosen the skins. When cool enough to handle, peel and seed the peppers. Dice the peppers.

In a small skillet, heat the oil and slowly sauté the onion and garlic until yellowed and soft, 5 minutes. Do not brown. In a cup, stir the sugar and salt into the vinegar until dissolved.

In a bowl, combine the oil, onion, garlic, bell peppers, and vinegar mixture. Season with freshly ground pepper to taste. Chill until needed, but bring to room temperature before using.

Kilocalories 90 Kc • Protein 1 gm • Fat 7 gm • Percent of calories from fat 66% • Cholesterol 0 mg • Dietary fiber 1 gm • Sodium 99 mg • Calcium 10 mg

Sicilian Eggplant Caponata

◼

MAKES 1 QUART, 8 APPETIZER SERVINGS

This Sicilian appetizer shows an Arab influence in the addition of golden raisins and vitamin E–rich nuts. Leftovers, if any, make a terrific lunch.

1 large eggplant (1¼ to 1½ pounds)
2 tablespoons olive oil, or more as needed
½ red bell pepper, seeded and diced
½ green bell pepper, seeded and diced
2 garlic cloves, minced
2 cups peeled seeded chopped fresh or undrained canned tomatoes
⅓ cup pitted black olives
⅓ cup pitted Sicilian green olives

¼ cup golden raisins
1 tablespoon drained capers
1 teaspoon chopped fresh oregano or ½ teaspoon dried
¼ teaspoon salt
¼ teaspoon freshly ground black pepper
3 tablespoons red wine vinegar
2 teaspoons sugar
¼ cup slivered almonds or toasted pine nuts
1 tablespoon minced fresh flat-leaf parsley
1 loaf French bread, sliced

Peel and slice the eggplant. Salt the slices and allow them to drain for a half hour or so. Rinse the slices and press them dry between paper towels. Dice the eggplant.

Heat the oil in a 12-inch skillet and sauté the peppers for 3 minutes. Add the eggplant and stir-fry over fairly high heat until it begins to turn color and soften, 5 to 8 minutes. This will use less oil than slower frying, but add more oil as you need it. During the last minute of frying, add the garlic, which should not brown.

Add the tomatoes, olives, raisins, capers, oregano, salt, and pepper, and simmer the mixture, uncovered, stirring often, until the sauce is thick and the vegetables are very tender but still retain their shape, 30 to 40 minutes. If using fresh tomatoes that aren't very juicy, add a little water as needed.

When the vegetables are cooked, add the vinegar and sugar, and stir to dissolve the sugar. Simmer 3 minutes. Taste to see if you want more vinegar or sugar.

Stir in the nuts and parsley. Serve at room temperature with small slices of crusty French bread.

Kilocalories 142 Kc • Protein 3 gm • Fat 8 gm • Percent of calories from fat 44% • Cholesterol 0 mg • Dietary fiber 5 gm • Sodium 228 mg • Calcium 32 mg

Corn and Black Bean Salsa

MAKES ABOUT 1 QUART, 8 SERVINGS

Serve this hearty salsa with nonfat or low-fat tortilla chips . . . or spoon some in a pita pocket for a vegetarian sandwich.

2 cups fresh or frozen corn kernels, or 1 (15-ounce) can corn kernels, drained

2 cups homemade black beans (page 16) or 1 (15- to 16-ounce) can low-sodium black beans, drained and rinsed

1 large or 2 small plum tomatoes, seeded and diced

½ cup finely chopped red onion

1 garlic clove, crushed through a press

1 Anaheim chili, seeded and diced

1 jalapeño chili, seeded and minced (wear rubber gloves)

¼ cup fresh lime juice or red wine vinegar

1 teaspoon ground cumin

½ teaspoon salt

¼ teaspoon freshly ground black pepper

2 tablespoons minced fresh cilantro

Simmer the corn kernels in water to cover for 3 minutes. (If using canned corn kernels, skip this step.) Drain and rinse in cold water. Combine the corn with all the remaining ingredients. Blend well so that the garlic and chilies are evenly distributed throughout. Chill several hours or overnight. Stir the salsa a few times while it's being chilled.

Kilocalories 81 Kc • Protein 4 gm • Fat 1 gm • Percent of calories from fat 6% • Cholesterol 0 mg • Dietary fiber 3 gm • Sodium 151 mg • Calcium 20 mg

Marinated Cauliflower

■

Lightly cooked vegetables make a nice change on the appetizer table.

1 large head cauliflower,
  separated into florets
¾ cup Garlic and Lemon
  Vinaigrette (page 19)

Hot red pepper flakes

Cut any large florets in half. You should have at least 15. Cook the cauliflower in boiling salted water until tender-crisp, about 3 minutes. Drain and rinse with cold water.

    Gently toss the cauliflower with the vinaigrette, adding hot red pepper flakes to taste. Chill. Serve as an appetizer with food picks or small forks.

Kilocalories 312 Kc • Protein 2 gm • Fat 33 gm • Percent of calories from fat 90% • Cholesterol 0 mg • Dietary fiber 2 gm • Sodium 112 mg • Calcium 23 mg

Sweet-and-Sour Sicilian Vegetables

To cut carrots safely, shave a little off one side so that the carrot will lie flat and not roll.

½ pound fresh green beans

2 large carrots, cut into sticks

1 (9-ounce) package frozen artichoke hearts

1 green bell pepper, seeded and cut into strips

4 tablespoons extra-virgin olive oil

4 scallions with green tops, chopped

2 to 3 tablespoons red wine vinegar

1 teaspoon sugar

¼ teaspoon salt

1 tablespoon finely chopped fresh mint

Freshly ground black pepper

Italian bread slices, quartered, as an accompaniment

Trim off the ends and cut the green beans diagonally into 2-inch pieces. Cook the green beans in boiling water until tender-crisp, about 5 minutes. Remove with a slotted spoon and rinse in cool water. Cook the carrots in the same water for 1 minute. Drain and rinse in cool water.

Cook the artichokes according to package directions. Rinse in cool water. If the artichokes are whole, cut them in half. In a small skillet, sauté the bell pepper in 1 tablespoon of oil until it's tender-crisp, 3 minutes.

In a shallow serving dish, combine the artichokes, green beans, carrots, bell pepper, and scallions. Dress the vegetables with the remaining 3 table-spoons of oil, the vinegar, sugar, salt, and mint, tossing to dissolve the sugar and salt. Add pepper to taste. Marinate at room temperature for a half hour or so. Taste to correct the seasoning; you may want more vinegar or sugar. Serve with small plates, forks, and hunks of crusty bread.

Kilocalories 198 Kc • Protein 4 gm • Fat 14 gm • Percent of calories from fat 59% • Cholesterol 0 mg • Dietary fiber 7 gm • Sodium 222 mg • Calcium 73 mg

APPETIZERS AND SNACKS

35

Antipasto Salad

■

Serve as an appetizer, or arrange the antipasto on lettuce leaves for a superlight luncheon dish.

2 cups homemade soybeans
   or chickpeas (page 16) or
   1 (14- to 16-ounce) can low-
   sodium soybeans or chickpeas,
   drained and rinsed
½ green bell pepper, seeded and
   chopped
½ red bell pepper, seeded and
   chopped
1 cup chopped fennel or celery
1 small carrot, very thinly
   sliced

¼ cup chopped sweet onion
½ pound fresh mozzarella, diced
1 (4-ounce) can pitted black
   olives, drained
¼ cup slivered oil-packed
   drained sun-dried tomatoes
½ cup or more Garlic and
   Lemon Vinaigrette (page 19)
Italian bread slices, quartered,
   as an accompaniment

Mix together the soybeans or chickpeas, bell pepper, fennel, carrot, onion, cheese, olives, and sun-dried tomatoes. Toss with the dressing. Marinate at room temperature for a half hour. Taste to determine if you want more dressing. Serve with small plates, forks, and hunks of crusty bread.

Kilocalories 410 Kc • Protein 23 gm • Fat 30 gm • Percent of calories from fat 62% • Cholesterol 11 mg • Dietary fiber 4 gm • Sodium 316 mg • Calcium 366 mg

Crabmeat-stuffed Cherry Tomatoes

■

These morsels look very pretty in their nest of dark green watercress— and they disappear fast.

1 bunch watercress
1 cup fresh or frozen thawed crabmeat, or 1 (6½-ounce) can crabmeat
2 teaspoons fresh lemon juice
1 pint firm unblemished cherry tomatoes (18 to 20)

1 tablespoon mayonnaise
1 tablespoon nonfat plain yogurt
1 teaspoon chopped fresh chives
1 teaspoon chopped fresh parsley
Few dashes of white pepper
Few dashes of cayenne

Wash and spin dry the watercress. Remove the tougher stems and cut the bunch in half to make smaller sprigs. Make a bed of watercress on a platter, cover with plastic wrap, and keep refrigerated until needed.

Flake the crabmeat; remove and discard any cartilage. Sprinkle it with the lemon juice. Cut off the tops of the cherry tomatoes, hollow them out (a grapefruit spoon works well for this task), and turn them upside down to drain while preparing the filling.

Whisk together the mayonnaise, yogurt, chives, and parsley. Add white pepper and cayenne to taste. Blend this dressing into the crabmeat. Turn the tomatoes right side up. Stuff them with the crabmeat mixture and nest the tomatoes on the prepared watercress bed. Chill until needed.

Kilocalories 66 Kc • Protein 8 gm • Fat 2 gm • Percent of calories from fat 32% • Cholesterol 24 mg • Dietary fiber 1 gm • Sodium 157 mg • Calcium 52 mg

LOBSTER-STUFFED CHERRY TOMATOES: Follow the preceding recipe, using 1 cup cooked, *very* finely diced lobster meat in place of the crabmeat. Substitute ½ teaspoon chopped fresh tarragon for the chives.

Kilocalories 66 Kc • Protein 8 gm • Fat 2 gm • Percent of calories from fat 32% • Cholesterol 37 mg • Dietary fiber 1 gm • Sodium 140 mg • Calcium 54 mg

SALMON-STUFFED CHERRY TOMATOES: Follow the preceding recipe, using 1 cup fresh cooked or 1 (8-ounce) can salmon in place of the crabmeat. Substitute 1 teaspoon chopped fresh dill for the parsley.

Kilocalories 69 Kc • Protein 8 gm • Fat 3 gm • Percent of calories from fat 38% • Cholesterol 22 mg • Dietary fiber 1 gm • Sodium 45 mg • Calcium 45 mg

Walnut 'n Wheat-stuffed Mushrooms

■

MAKES 4 SERVINGS

If you can't find very large mushrooms, you can use 1 pound of medium-large just as well. They may cook in slightly less time.

8 large "stuffing" mushrooms, cleaned (about 1 pound)
2 tablespoons olive oil, plus more for drizzling on top
1 garlic clove, minced
1 cup fresh bread crumbs made from 1 slice Italian bread
½ cup finely chopped walnuts
2 tablespoons toasted wheat germ

1 tablespoon grated Parmesan cheese, plus more for sprinkling
1 teaspoon chopped fresh thyme or ¼ teaspoon dried
⅛ teaspoon freshly ground black pepper

Remove the mushroom stems and chop them into a fine dice. Heat the oil in a medium skillet, and sauté the mushroom stems over medium-high heat, stirring often, until they begin to brown, 3 to 5 minutes. Lower the heat and add the garlic, blending well. Cook 1 minute more. Add the bread crumbs and stir-fry until they are golden, about 1 minute. Remove from the heat and stir in the walnuts, wheat germ, cheese, thyme, and pepper. Add a tablespoon or more of water to moisten the stuffing just enough to hold together when pressed.

Stuff the mushroom caps with the mixture and put them into an oiled baking dish. Drizzle a little more oil on top and sprinkle with a teaspoon or so of cheese. If any stuffing is left over, you can sprinkle it around the mushrooms.

The mushrooms can be made ahead to this point. If held over an hour, refrigerate them.

When ready to cook, preheat the oven to 350 degrees F. Bake the mushrooms for 20 minutes, or until they are tender and golden brown.

Kilocalories 223 Kc • Protein 8 gm • Fat 17 gm • Percent of calories from fat 64% • Cholesterol 1 mg • Dietary fiber 3 gm • Sodium 72 mg • Calcium 44 mg

Bruschetta with Broccoli de Rabe

MAKES 8 SLICES

When you prepare this recipe, some broccoli de rabe may be left over. If so, it makes a nice addition to soup.

1 bunch broccoli de rabe (about ¾ pound)
2 tablespoons olive oil
2 garlic cloves, minced
½ cup chicken or vegetable stock (pages 10, 11) or low-sodium canned broth

8 slices Italian bread
8 tablespoons freshly grated Parmesan cheese
1 to 2 roasted red peppers (from a jar), cut into strips (optional)

Wash the broccoli de rabe well and trim off the tough stems. Heat 1 tablespoon of the oil in a 10-inch skillet and sauté the garlic until it sizzles, about 1 minute. Add the broccoli de rabe and stock, cover, and simmer until the broccoli de rabe is tender, about 10 minutes. Drain well, including as much of the garlic as possible with the broccoli de rabe. Press out excess moisture with the back of a spoon. Chop the broccoli de rabe to a fine texture.

Toast the bread on one side under a broiler. Remove the slices. Brush them with the remaining tablespoon of oil. Spread about 2 tablespoons of broccoli de rabe on each, sprinkle with a tablespoon of the cheese, and decorate with strips of roasted red pepper.

Put the slices on a baking pan and broil them 6 inches from the heat source until the cheese is melted and the edges of the bread are golden, 1 to 2 minutes. Serve hot.

Kilocalories 312 Kc • Protein 12 gm • Fat 12 gm • Percent of calories from fat 35% • Cholesterol 8 mg • Dietary fiber 2 gm • Sodium 558 mg • Calcium 340 mg

BRUSCHETTA WITH SPINACH AND ANCHOVIES: Follow the preceding recipe, substituting 10 ounces spinach for the broccoli de rabe. Cook only until wilted. Omit the roasted red pepper strips and garnish each slice instead with a vinegar-rinsed anchovy fillet.

Kilocalories 307 Kc • Protein 14 gm • Fat 13 gm • Percent of calories from fat 37% • Cholesterol 15 mg • Dietary fiber 4 gm • Sodium 818 mg • Calcium 276 mg

BRUSCHETTA WITH TOMATO AND PROVOLONE:

2 cups unpeeled seeded chopped plum tomatoes (about 6)	2 tablespoons olive oil
	Salt
1 garlic clove, crushed through a press	8 slices Italian bread
	About 4 slices provolone cheese, cut into 16 strips
2 fresh basil leaves, slivered	

Mix together the tomatoes, garlic, basil, oil, and salt to taste, keeping in mind that the provolone is salty. Allow the mixture to marinate for 30 minutes or more at room temperature.

Toast the bread on one side under a broiler. Remove the slices. Divide the tomato mixture between the slices of bread. Garnish each with 2 strips of provolone cheese.

Put the slices on a baking pan and broil them 6 inches from the heat source until the cheese is melted and the edges of the bread are golden, 1 to 2 minutes. Serve hot.

Kilocalories 326 Kc • Protein 15 gm • Fat 13 gm • Percent of calories from fat 36% • Cholesterol 17 mg • Dietary fiber 3 gm • Sodium 500 mg • Calcium 254 mg

BRUSCHETTA WITH CHILIES: This version has lots of zing! Follow the preceding recipe, adding 1 to 2 minced canned jalapeño chilies (if you handle them, wear rubber gloves) to the tomatoes. Substitute 8 tablespoons (½ cup) coarsely grated Monterey Jack cheese for the provolone, 1 tablespoon for each portion.

Kilocalories 298 Kc • Protein 9 gm • Fat 14 gm • Percent of calories from fat 41% • Cholesterol 15 mg • Dietary fiber 3 gm • Sodium 509 mg • Calcium 154 mg

Broccoli Squares

Everyone seems to love these tasty squares, and this easy recipe makes a lot of them!

½ pound broccoli crowns
1 large garlic clove, unpeeled
4 eggs or 1 cup egg substitute
½ cup vegetable oil
1 tablespoon chopped fresh
  parsley
¼ teaspoon dried oregano
¼ teaspoon dried basil

¼ teaspoon salt
⅛ teaspoon cayenne
1 cup unbleached
  all-purpose flour
½ teaspoon baking powder
¼ cup chopped sweet onion
½ cup grated Parmesan cheese

Preheat the oven to 375 degrees F. Oil a 13 × 9-inch baking pan.

Cut the broccoli into florets with ½-inch stems. Parboil the broccoli and garlic in boiling salted water for 3 minutes, counting the time from when the water boils again after adding the broccoli. Cool slightly and chop the broccoli. You should have about 3 cups; a little less is okay. Mince the garlic.

Beat together the eggs, oil, parsley, oregano, basil, salt, and cayenne. Whisk in the flour and baking powder. Stir in the onion, cheese, and garlic. Fold in the broccoli. Pour the batter into the prepared pan.

Bake until golden brown, about 25 minutes. Cool slightly and cut into 2-inch squares to serve.

Kilocalories 248 Kc • Protein 8 gm • Fat 18 gm • Percent of calories from fat 64% • Cholesterol 110 mg • Dietary fiber 1 gm • Sodium 230 mg • Calcium 112 mg

APPETIZERS AND SNACKS

Melon Platter with Smoked Salmon

———————————— ■ ————————————

MAKES **8** SERVINGS

This appetizer is about as simple as it gets—but it's lovely to look at and a delicious combination.

1 cantaloupe
½ small honeydew melon
1 pound smoked salmon, thinly
   sliced

Freshly ground black pepper
Lemon and lime wedges

Peel and seed the melons. Slice in ½-inch slices. Arrange overlapping slices of cantaloupe, honeydew, and salmon on a platter. Season with a few grinds of pepper. Garnish with lemon and lime wedges.

Kilocalories 138 Kc • Protein 12 gm • Fat 3 gm • Percent of calories from fat 17% • Cholesterol 13 mg • Dietary fiber 2 gm • Sodium 482 mg • Calcium 30 mg

Soups and Chowders

A dish for all seasons, soup is the most adaptable of foods. In winter, you can simmer a heartwarming Barley and Vegetable Soup. In spring, Asparagus and New Potato Chowder with Tarragon will lend a seasonal flair to the table. In summer, a Chilled Peach and Lime Soup is sure to whet the wilted appetite. And when autumn arrives, it's time to enjoy a tempting Halloween Pumpkin and Apple Soup.

Many of the recipes in this chapter call for stock as an ingredient. These homemade chicken or vegetable broths make easy preparation possible by adding long-cooked flavor to a quick soup. Recipes for homemade stocks are given in the Basics chapter. But if you don't have the time or inclination to make stocks, keep several cans of a low-sodium canned broth on hand instead—for those moments when you're inspired to make a beautiful antioxidant-rich soup. Vegetable broth, as well as chicken, is generally available on supermarket shelves.

Bean soups are among the most nutritious and comforting of soups. You can make them with Homemade Beans (page 16) or for convenience, use canned beans. Many varieties—big or small, dark or light, chewy or soft—are available at your local supermarket. But it's even better to seek out a natural food store that sells organic, low-sodium or no-salt-added canned beans. Canned soybeans, the one bean that's not readily found in supermarkets, are stocked in many natural food stores.

Soup is a terrific way to add good nutrition to the daily fare, since most of its traditional ingredients are important antioxidant foods. Even people who are fussy about their veggies can find them quite palatable in a savory or creamy broth.

Depending on the ingredients, the season, and whatever else will be included in the meal, soup can be a luncheon dish, a first course, or the main event. A good fresh bakery bread and a complementary salad will often be all that is needed to accompany a substantial soup—such as Lentil and Pasta Soup with Balsamic Vinegar or Salmon, Corn, and Zucchini Chowder—for one of the easiest homestyle meals you can create on a busy day. Enjoy!

Asparagus and New Potato Chowder with Tarragon

Here's a taste of spring! Fresh Salmon and Watercress Salad (page 149) and light rye bread would round out a lovely seasonal menu.

12 whole baby red potatoes, unpeeled (¾ pound)

¾ pound fresh asparagus

6 scallions, chopped

5 cups chicken stock (page 10) or canned low-sodium broth

¼ cup nonfat dry milk powder

2 tablespoons superfine flour, such as Wondra

¼ teaspoon salt

⅛ to ¼ teaspoon white pepper

1 cup low-fat milk

2 teaspoons chopped fresh tarragon or ½ teaspoon dried

Scrub the potatoes well, removing any little sprouts or black marks, and leave them unpeeled. Steam the potatoes until they are tender, about 15 minutes. Cut them in half.

Wash the asparagus, remove the woody ends and chop the stalks; reserve the tips. In a large pot, combine the asparagus stalks, scallions, and stock. Simmer until the asparagus is quite tender, 10 minutes. Puree the soup in batches. Return it to the pot. Add the asparagus tips and potatoes, and simmer until the tips are tender-crisp, about 3 minutes.

Whisk the dry milk, flour, salt, and pepper to taste (¼ teaspoon will make the soup quite peppery) into the liquid milk. Add all at once to the simmering soup, and stir constantly until the soup bubbles and thickens slightly, about 5 minutes. Reduce the heat, add the tarragon, and simmer over low heat for 3 minutes, stirring often.

Kilocalories 144 Kc • Protein 7 gm • Fat 1 gm • Percent of calories from fat 10% • Cholesterol 4 mg • Dietary fiber 3 gm • Sodium 164 mg • Calcium 86 mg

Navy Bean Soup with Parsley Pesto

This from-scratch soup has to be started a day ahead, but it's worth the time.

2 cups dried navy beans, rinsed and picked over
2 tablespoons olive oil
1 large yellow onion, chopped
1 celery stalk with leaves, diced
2 garlic cloves, minced
9 cups vegetable or chicken stock (pages 11, 10) or canned low-sodium broth
¼ cup low-sodium tomato paste

1 teaspoon chopped fresh rosemary or ¼ teaspoon dried
1 teaspoon chopped fresh sage or ¼ teaspoon dried leaves (not ground)
Salt (optional)
Freshly ground black pepper
About ½ cup Parsley Pesto (page 14)

Put the beans in a large pot with 2 quarts water and soak them overnight in a cool place. The next day, drain and rinse the beans.

In the same pot, heat the olive oil and sauté the onion, celery, and garlic for 3 minutes. Add the stock, tomato paste, rosemary, sage, and drained beans. Simmer the beans until tender, about 2 hours.

Remove 1 cup cooked beans with a slotted spoon and mash them or puree in a food processor. Return the mashed beans to the soup. Taste to correct the seasoning. The reduced stock should be salty enough, but you may want more. Add freshly ground pepper to taste. Swirl a spoonful of parsley pesto into each serving.

Kilocalories 464 Kc • Protein 20 gm • Fat 17 gm • Percent of calories from fat 31% • Cholesterol 0 mg • Dietary fiber 19 gm • Sodium 153 mg • Calcium 146 mg

Kidney Bean Soup with Fresh Herbs

MAKES 4 SERVINGS

Fresh herbs retain their color and flavor better if you add them at the end of the cooking time. Dried herbs should be added earlier.

2 tablespoons olive oil
2 cups finely diced carrots
1 large onion, chopped
4 or more cups vegetable or chicken stock (pages 11, 10) or canned low-sodium broth
3½ cups homemade kidney beans (page 16) or 2 (14- to 16-ounce) cans low-sodium kidney beans, drained and rinsed

¼ teaspoon freshly ground black pepper
2 tablespoons chopped fresh flat-leaf parsley
2 tablespoons chopped fresh chives

Heat the oil in a large pot and sauté the carrots and onion until lightly colored, 5 minutes. Add the stock and beans. Bring to a simmer and cook, covered, for 15 minutes. Puree the soup in batches in a food processor and return it to the pan. If the soup seems too thick, add more stock. Reheat and stir in the pepper, parsley, and chives.

Kilocalories 359 Kc • Protein 18 gm • Fat 8 gm • Percent of calories from fat 19% • Cholesterol 0 mg • Dietary fiber 19 gm • Sodium 79 mg • Calcium 121 mg

SOUPS AND CHOWDERS

Black Bean Soup with Chopped Tomatoes

The popular combination of black beans and corn appears here in another guise. I like plenty of pepper in this one!

1 cup peeled seeded chopped
  tomatoes
½ cup chopped scallions
3 tablespoons olive oil
Dash of salt
2 cups finely diced carrots
1 large onion, chopped
5 cups or more vegetable or
  chicken stock (pages 11, 10) or
  canned low-sodium broth
3½ cups homemade black beans
  (page 16) or 2 (14- to 16-
  ounce) cans low-sodium black
  beans, drained and rinsed

1 cup fresh or frozen corn
  kernels
¼ teaspoon freshly ground black
  pepper
⅛ teaspoon cayenne (optional)
2 tablespoons chopped fresh
  cilantro

In a small bowl, toss the tomatoes and scallions with 1 tablespoon of the oil and the salt. Let the mixture marinate at room temperature while making the soup.

Heat the remaining 2 tablespoons of oil in a large pot and sauté the carrots and onion until lightly colored, 5 minutes. Add the stock and beans. Bring to a simmer and cook, covered, for 15 minutes. Puree the soup in batches in a food processor and return it to the pan. If the soup seems too thick, add more stock.

Stir in the corn, black pepper, cayenne, and cilantro, and cook over very low heat, stirring often, for 5 minutes. Serve in shallow soup bowls and garnish each serving with a spoonful of chopped tomatoes.

Kilocalories 450 Kc • Protein 18 gm • Fat 12 gm • Percent of calories from fat 22% • Cholesterol 0 mg • Dietary fiber 14 gm • Sodium 85 mg • Calcium 119 mg

Curried Red Lentil Soup

MAKES 4 SERVINGS

After cooking, red lentils don't retain their lovely color, but they cook faster and have a different, milder flavor than brown lentils.

2 tablespoons canola oil
1 large onion, chopped
4 carrots, chopped
1 garlic clove, minced
2 teaspoons mild curry powder
½ teaspoon ground cumin
¼ teaspoon ground cinnamon

1 cup red lentils, picked over,
  rinsed and drained
5 cups vegetable stock (page 11)
  or canned low-sodium broth
1 tablespoon chopped fresh
  cilantro leaves or fresh chives

Heat the oil in a large heavy saucepan and sauté the onion and carrots until they are lightly colored, about 5 minutes. Stir in the garlic, curry, cumin, and cinnamon. Sauté 1 minute longer. Add the lentils and stock. Simmer the soup, covered, stirring often, until everything is quite tender, about 25 minutes. Puree the soup in batches and return to the pot to rewarm. Stir in the cilantro or chives.

Kilocalories 324 Kc • Protein 16 gm • Fat 8 gm • Percent of calories from fat 22% • Cholesterol 0 mg • Dietary fiber 18 gm • Sodium 85 mg • Calcium 66 mg

SOUPS AND CHOWDERS

Lentil and Pasta Soup with Balsamic Vinegar

MAKES **8** SERVINGS

This is a popular and hearty soup for those times when you need a lot of easy food, such as Super Bowl Sunday.

1 pound brown lentils
2 tablespoons olive oil
1 large yellow onion, chopped
2 celery stalks, chopped
3 garlic cloves, finely chopped
1 cup sliced carrots (small slices)
6 cups vegetable or chicken stock (pages 11, 10) or canned low-sodium broth

1 teaspoon dried Italian herbs (or a combination of dried oregano, basil, thyme, and rosemary)
¼ teaspoon freshly ground black pepper
¼ cup balsamic vinegar
Salt (optional)
1 cup ditalini (small pasta tubes)

Pick over and rinse the lentils. In a large heavy pot, heat the oil and sauté the onion, celery, and garlic until softened but not brown, about 3 minutes. Add the lentils, carrots, stock, 4 cups water, and herbs. Bring to a boil and simmer the soup with the cover slightly ajar, stirring often (especially at the end of the cooking time), until the lentils are very tender but still retain their shape, 45 to 50 minutes. Stir in the pepper and vinegar. Taste the soup and add salt if you wish.

If making the soup ahead of time, stop at this point. Cool and refrigerate the soup. Add a little stock or low-sodium broth when reheating. Add the pasta just before serving so that it won't soak up all the broth.

When ready to serve, cook the ditalini separately according to package directions. Drain. Stir into the soup.

Kilocalories 332 Kc • Protein 20 gm • Fat 5 gm • Percent of calories from fat 12% • Cholesterol 0 mg • Dietary fiber 18 gm • Sodium 58 mg • Calcium 55 mg

Broccoli and Rice Chowder

Broccoli's become a popular soup flavor, recently added to the repertoire of commercial brands. But if you compare prices, you'll see you can make a whole pot of homemade soup for the cost of one can of supermarket soup.

½ pound broccoli crowns
5 cups chicken stock (page 10)
  or canned low-sodium broth
6 scallions, chopped
½ cup nonfat dry milk powder
5 tablespoons superfine flour,
  such as Wondra

¼ teaspoon salt
¼ teaspoon white pepper
2 cups low-fat milk
2½ cups cooked long-grain
  white rice
½ cup chopped roasted red bell
  pepper (from a jar—optional)

Chop the broccoli into small pieces; you should have 2½ to 3 cups.

Bring the stock to a boil in a large pot. Add the broccoli and scallions, and simmer for 5 minutes, or until the vegetables are tender.

Whisk the dry milk, flour, salt, and pepper into the liquid milk. Add all at once to the simmering soup, and stir constantly until the soup bubbles and thickens slightly, about 5 minutes. Reduce the heat to low and simmer for 3 minutes, stirring often. Add the rice and roasted red pepper, if using, and cook 2 minutes longer. Taste to determine if you want more salt or pepper.

Kilocalories 255 Kc • Protein 10 gm • Fat 2 gm • Percent of calories from fat 9% • Cholesterol 7 mg • Dietary fiber 2 gm • Sodium 196 mg • Calcium 158 mg

SOUPS AND CHOWDERS

51

Sweet-and-Sour Green Cabbage Soup

■

MAKES 6 SERVINGS

Here's a very low-fat but substantial soup. Fresh rye bread is a naturally nice accompaniment.

7 cups chicken stock (page 10) or canned low-sodium broth (see Note)

3 tablespoons low-sodium tomato paste

4 cups coarsely chopped green cabbage (½ large head)

¼ teaspoon salt

2 tablespoons balsamic vinegar

2 teaspoons dark brown sugar

1 tablespoon chopped fresh cilantro or 1 teaspoon dried

⅛ to ¼ teaspoon freshly ground black pepper

1 cup cooked brown rice

Combine the stock, tomato paste, cabbage, and salt in a large pot. Bring to a boil and simmer, covered, until the cabbage is tender, about 8 minutes. Stir in the vinegar, brown sugar, cilantro, pepper, and rice. Continue cooking over very low heat for 3 minutes. Taste to correct the seasoning, adding more vinegar or sugar to taste.

NOTE: To produce a fat-free stock, chill the stock until the fat gels; remove the fat with a slotted spoon.

Kilocalories 115 Kc • Protein 5 gm • Fat 1 gm • Percent of calories from fat 9% • Cholesterol 2 mg • Dietary fiber 2 gm • Sodium 161 mg • Calcium 28 mg

Carrot and Caraway Soup

There's lots of beta-carotene in every bowlful of this soup.

1 tablespoon olive oil
2 leeks, well washed, chopped
1 pound carrots, sliced
About 4 cups chicken or
  vegetable stock (pages 10, 11)
  or canned low-sodium broth

¼ teaspoon white pepper
½ teaspoon caraway seeds,
  crushed in a mortar with pestle

Heat the oil in a large saucepan and "sweat" the leeks over very low heat for 10 minutes. Add the carrots and continue sautéing for 5 minutes; the vegetables should be golden but not brown. Add 2 cups stock or broth. Simmer, covered, until the vegetables are very tender, about 30 minutes.

Puree the soup in batches in a food processor. Return the puree to the pan. Add enough broth to make a creamy soup thickness to your taste. Stir in the pepper and caraway seeds. Keep the soup warm for 5 minutes or so to develop the flavor.

Kilocalories 158 Kc • Protein 5 gm • Fat 4 gm • Percent of calories from fat 26% • Cholesterol 2 mg • Dietary fiber 5 gm • Sodium 94 mg • Calcium 69 mg

Carrot Vichyssoise

This is a make-ahead, pleasing starter for a summer supper.

3 tablespoons olive oil
2 to 3 large leeks (1 bunch), well washed, chopped
2 celery stalks with leaves, chopped
4 cups peeled chopped potatoes
2 cups chopped carrots
6 cups chicken stock (page 10) or canned low-sodium broth
1 tablespoon lemon juice
1 tablespoon chopped fresh dill or 1 teaspoon dried

¼ teaspoon salt, or more
1 cup nonfat plain yogurt
3 tablespoons finely chopped fresh chives or ¼ cup finely chopped green scallion tops
¼ teaspoon white pepper, or more
Additional fresh dill or chives for garnish (optional)

In a large pot, heat the oil and slowly sauté the leeks and celery stalks over very low heat until they are very soft but not brown. Add the potatoes, carrots, stock, lemon juice, dill, and salt, and simmer until the vegetables are very tender, about 30 minutes. Cool the soup. Puree it in batches in a food processor; return the soup to the pot. Blend in the yogurt, chives, and white pepper. Taste to correct the seasoning, adding more salt and/or pepper as desired. Chill the soup. Serve cold, garnished with sprigs of fresh chive or dill, if you wish.

Kilocalories 292 Kc • Protein 10 gm • Fat 8 gm • Percent of calories from fat 24% • Cholesterol 2 mg • Dietary fiber 5 gm • Sodium 210 mg • Calcium 128 mg

Corn Chowder with Broccoli

A 5-star green vegetable enriches this old-fashioned favorite.

1 tablespoon butter
1 small onion, chopped
2 cups fresh broccoli, cut into
  small florets and ½-inch slices
  of stalk
2 medium potatoes, peeled
  and diced
2 cups fresh or frozen corn, or
  1 (15-ounce) can low-sodium
  creamed corn

¼ teaspoon salt
2½ cups low-fat milk
2 tablespoons superfine flour,
  such as Wondra
1 teaspoon chopped fresh thyme
  or ¼ teaspoon dried
Several dashes of white pepper
Cayenne (optional)

Melt the butter in a large saucepan and sauté the onion until it's soft and yellow, 3 to 5 minutes. Add the broccoli, potatoes, fresh or frozen corn (if you're using creamed corn, add it when the vegetables are cooked), 1 cup water, and salt. Cover and simmer the vegetables until tender, 5 minutes. Add 2 cups of the milk (and creamed corn, if using) and heat but do not boil until you've added the thickener.

Blend the flour into the remaining ½ cup milk, add it to the chowder, and cook over medium heat, stirring constantly, until the chowder bubbles and thickens, about 5 minutes. Add the thyme and white pepper to taste. Simmer over very low heat, stirring often, for 3 minutes. If desired, top each serving with a dash of cayenne.

Kilocalories 396 Kc • Protein 15 gm • Fat 7 gm • Percent of calories from fat 14% • Cholesterol 20 mg • Dietary fiber 7 gm • Sodium 286 mg • Calcium 237 mg

Eggplant Soup Provençal

■

Versatile eggplant makes a "creamy" (without cream) and flavorful soup.

1 eggplant (about 1 pound)
Salt
2 tablespoons olive oil, plus
  more if needed
1 medium onion, chopped
1 garlic clove, chopped
1 cup peeled chopped fresh or
  undrained canned tomatoes
Several fresh basil leaves,
  chopped, or ½ teaspoon dried

3 cups vegetable or chicken
  stock (pages 11, 10) or canned
  low-sodium broth
¼ cup nonfat dry milk powder
2 tablespoons cornstarch
Freshly ground black pepper
1 cup low-fat milk
¼ cup chopped fresh flat-leaf
  parsley for garnish

Peel and dice the eggplant. Sprinkle with salt and allow it to drain in a colander for a half hour or so. Rinse well and press dry between paper towels.

Heat the oil in a large skillet, and stir-fry the eggplant, onion, and garlic for 5 to 8 minutes, until softened but not brown. Add the tomatoes and basil. Cover and simmer over low heat until the eggplant is very tender, about 15 minutes.

Puree the eggplant in a food processor or blender, adding 1 cup of the stock. Pour the puree into a saucepan and whisk in the remaining 2 cups stock. Simmer the soup for 5 minutes.

Whisk the dry milk, cornstarch, ¼ teaspoon salt, and pepper to taste into the liquid milk. Pour into the simmering soup, and stir constantly until the mixture boils again and thickens slightly, about 2 minutes. Simmer 2 to 3 minutes more, stirring often. Garnish each portion with chopped parsley.

Kilocalories 195 Kc • Protein 5 gm • Fat 9 gm • Percent of calories from fat 38% • Cholesterol 5 mg • Dietary fiber 4 gm • Sodium 224 mg • Calcium 113 mg

Kale Soup with Sweet and Yellow Potatoes

———————————■———————————

MAKES 6 SERVINGS

Sautéing onion and garlic in oil gives a flavorful base to this soup. A round loaf of Portuguese bread makes an ideal accompaniment.

1 bunch kale (about ¾ pound)
2 tablespoons olive oil
1 large yellow onion, diced
2 garlic cloves, chopped
1 pound sweet potatoes, peeled and diced
1 pound yellow potatoes, such as Yukon Gold, peeled and diced

4 cups vegetable or chicken stock (pages 11, 10) or canned low-sodium broth
¼ teaspoon salt (optional)
⅛ to ¼ teaspoon freshly ground black pepper, to taste
½ cup slivered provolone cheese for garnish (optional)

Wash the kale well and remove the tough stems. Chop the leaves roughly into 2-inch pieces.

In a large pot, heat the oil and sauté the onion until it's lightly colored, about 3 minutes. Add the garlic and sauté 1 minute longer. Add the potatoes, kale, 2 cups water, and stock. Bring to a simmer, cover, and cook until the vegetables are quite tender, 20 to 25 minutes. Taste before adding salt. Stir in the pepper. Garnish each serving with a heaping tablespoon of slivered provolone cheese, if you wish.

Kilocalories 221 Kc • Protein 5 gm • Fat 5 gm • Percent of calories from fat 21% • Cholesterol 0 mg • Dietary fiber 5 gm • Sodium 57 mg • Calcium 82 mg

SOUPS AND CHOWDERS

57

Kale and Lentil Soup

———— ■ ————

Hearty kale keeps on growing when other greens fall victim to the cold weather. No wonder it's one of the top disease-fighting vegetables!

1 bunch kale (about ¾ pound)
2 tablespoons olive oil
1 cup chopped fennel or celery
1 cup chopped carrots
1 medium yellow onion, chopped
2 garlic cloves, chopped
6 cups vegetable or chicken stock (pages 11, 10) or canned low-sodium broth

1 cup brown lentils, rinsed and picked over
¼ teaspoon freshly ground black pepper
1 to 2 tablespoons balsamic vinegar, to taste
¼ teaspoon salt (optional)

Wash the kale well, trim off the tough stems, and chop it coarsely.

In a large pot, heat the oil and sauté the fennel or celery, carrots, onion, and garlic until yellowed, about 5 minutes. Add the stock, 1½ cups water, and lentils, bring to a boil, and reduce the heat until the soup is simmering. Cover and cook for 30 minutes. Add the kale, pepper, and vinegar, and continue cooking for 20 minutes. Stir occasionally during cooking. When the soup is ready, taste it to determine if you want to add the salt.

Kilocalories 238 Kc • Protein 12 gm • Fat 6 gm • Percent of calories from fat 21% • Cholesterol 0 mg • Dietary fiber 13 gm • Sodium 79 mg • Calcium 88 mg

ANTIOXIDANT POWER

58

Italian Spinach and Rice Soup

A good source of both beta-carotene and vitamin E, spinach doubles up on antioxidant power.

1 pound fresh spinach
2 tablespoons olive oil
5 ounces cleaned sliced
   mushrooms
6 cups chicken or vegetable
   stock (pages 10, 11) or canned
   low-sodium broth

½ cup arborio rice
¼ teaspoon salt (optional)
Freshly ground black pepper
Dash of ground nutmeg
Grated Parmesan cheese

Wash the spinach well and trim off the tough stems. Chop the spinach coarsely.

In a large pot, heat the oil and fry the mushrooms over medium-high heat until they are brown, about 5 minutes. Add the broth and rice. Bring the soup to a simmer, cover, and cook 15 minutes. Add the spinach and cook an additional 5 minutes. Season with salt, if needed (it depends on the stock or broth you've used), pepper to taste, and nutmeg. Pass the cheese at the table.

Kilocalories 161 Kc • Protein 7 gm • Fat 5 gm • Percent of calories from fat 33% • Cholesterol 2 mg • Dietary fiber 3 gm • Sodium 103 mg • Calcium 77 mg

Romaine Lettuce and Leek Soup

The distinctive flavor of leeks is especially pleasing in soups.

3 large leeks, white part only (1 bunch)
1 tablespoon olive oil
1 large head romaine lettuce, cored and coarsely chopped
1 large carrot, coarsely shredded
6 cups chicken or vegetable stock (pages 10, 11) or canned low-sodium broth
⅛ teaspoon freshly ground black pepper
¼ teaspoon salt (optional)
6 ounces fine egg noodles (about ⅓ pound)
2 tablespoons chopped fresh flat-leaf parsley
2 tablespoons lemon juice

Slice the leeks lengthwise and wash between the rings. Chop the leeks. Heat the oil in a large pot and "sweat" the leeks over very low heat until they are softened, lightly colored, and tender, 10 minutes.

Add the lettuce, carrot, stock, and pepper. Bring to a simmer, cover, and cook until the vegetables are quite tender, 8 to 10 minutes. Taste to determine if you need the salt.

Cook the egg noodles in a separate pot according to package directions, drain, and stir them into the soup. Add the parsley and lemon juice just before serving.

Kilocalories 222 Kc • Protein 9 gm • Fat 4 gm • Percent of calories from fat 18% • Cholesterol 28 mg • Dietary fiber 3 gm • Sodium 70 mg • Calcium 71 mg

ANTIOXIDANT POWER

Escarole and Carrot Soup with Pancetta

Italian bacon, called pancetta, is not smoked like American bacon. It's sold at many supermarket deli counters. Just a little pancetta will impart a delectable flavor to a whole pot of soup.

1 bunch escarole (about 1 pound)	2 large carrots, cut into ½-inch slices
2 slices pancetta, diced	Salt (optional)
1 tablespoon olive oil	Freshly ground black pepper
2 garlic cloves, minced	4 ounces thin egg noodles (¼ pound)
6 cups vegetable or chicken stock (pages 11, 10) or canned low-sodium broth	

Wash the escarole well and chop it coarsely.

In a large pot, fry the pancetta until it's brown and crisp. Remove the pancetta with a slotted spoon and discard the fat.

Heat the oil in the same pot and sauté the garlic until it's sizzling and fragrant but not brown, 2 minutes. Add the stock, escarole, and carrots. Add salt if needed (taste the stock to decide) and pepper to taste. Bring to a boil, cover, and simmer until the vegetables are tender, about 15 minutes. Return the pancetta to the soup pot.

Cook the noodles separately according to package directions and drain them. Stir them into the soup.

Kilocalories 174 Kc • Protein 7 gm • Fat 5 gm • Percent of calories from fat 23% • Cholesterol 23 mg • Dietary fiber 4 gm • Sodium 196 mg • Calcium 54 mg

SOUPS AND CHOWDERS

Peas and Chickpeas Soup

This soup is extra thick and hearty—and extra rich in antioxidants, too.

5 cups well-flavored chicken
   broth (homemade is ideal)
2 large carrots, diced
1 cup frozen peas
1 cup canned chickpeas, drained
   and rinsed
1 cup cooked brown rice, or any
   rice, or even leftover pasta

Freshly ground black pepper
Salt (optional)
1 tablespoon minced fresh
   parsley
Grated Parmesan cheese

In a large pot, combine the broth and carrots and bring to a boil. Reduce the heat and simmer until the carrots are nearly tender, about 8 minutes. Add the peas, chickpeas, and rice, with pepper to taste, and continue cooking for 5 minutes. Taste to determine if you need salt. Stir in the parsley and serve. Pass the cheese at the table.

Kilocalories 219 Kc • Protein 11 gm • Fat 2 gm • Percent of calories from fat 10% • Cholesterol 2 mg • Dietary fiber 7 gm • Sodium 104 mg • Calcium 46 mg

Riso con Piselli (Italian Rice and Peas Soup)

MAKES 4 SERVINGS

Bruschetta with Tomato and Provolone (page 40) would go well along-side this perfect luncheon soup.

1 (¼-inch) slice pancetta (Italian bacon) or 2 slices bacon (optional)

2 tablespoons olive oil

1 medium yellow onion, chopped

1 garlic clove, minced

6 cups vegetable or chicken stock (pages 11, 10) or canned low-sodium broth

½ cup arborio rice

1½ cups shelled fresh peas or 1 (10-ounce) package frozen peas

Freshly ground black pepper

Salt (optional)

1 tablespoon chopped fresh flat-leaf parsley

Freshly ground Parmesan cheese

Dice the pancetta (or bacon) and fry it until brown and crisp. Discard the fat. Drain the pancetta on a paper towel.

Heat the olive oil in a large pot. Sauté the onion until it's yellowed and limp, 3 to 5 minutes. Add the garlic in the last minute. Add the broth and rice. Simmer the soup, covered, for 15 minutes. Add the peas and simmer 5 minutes longer (counting the time from when the soup begins to bubble). Add pepper to taste; if adding pancetta, you may not need salt. Stir in the parsley and pancetta. Pass a dish of grated cheese at the table.

Kilocalories 274 Kc • Protein 7 gm • Fat 8 gm • Percent of calories from fat 25% • Cholesterol 0 mg • Dietary fiber 4 gm • Sodium 67 mg • Calcium 29 mg

Chilled Red Bell Pepper Soup with Basil

Here's a cool soup to start a summertime meal.

2 tablespoons olive oil
1 large yellow onion, chopped
4 large red bell peppers, seeded
 and cut into 1-inch chunks
½ cup dry vermouth or
 white wine
1 large potato, peeled and cut
 into 1-inch chunks

4 cups vegetable or chicken
 stock (pages 11, 10) or canned
 low-sodium broth
Freshly ground black pepper
Salt (optional)
1 cup nonfat plain yogurt
¼ cup slivered fresh basil

Heat the olive oil in a large pot, and sauté the onion and bell peppers until they're limp, about 5 minutes. Add the wine and continue cooking until it's reduced by half, about 2 minutes. Add the potato and stock. Simmer until the vegetables are very tender, about 20 minutes. Cool the soup slightly and puree it in batches in a food processor. Stir in the pepper. Taste to determine if you need salt. Chill the soup until it's completely cold. Just before serving, whisk in the yogurt and basil.

Kilocalories 195 Kc • Protein 5 gm • Fat 5 gm • Percent of calories from fat 22% • Cholesterol 0 mg • Dietary fiber 3 gm • Sodium 64 mg • Calcium 95 mg

ANTIOXIDANT POWER

Butternut-Tomato Soup

Double the antioxidant power when tomatoes and squash team up!

1 tablespoon olive oil

2 garlic cloves, minced

3 cups butternut squash cubes, peeled (about ¾ pound)

1 (1-pound) can tomatoes with juice

6 cups vegetable or chicken stock (pages 11, 10) or canned low-sodium broth

1 tablespoon chopped fresh dill or 1 teaspoon dried

¼ teaspoon celery salt

¼ teaspoon freshly ground black pepper

¼ cup nonfat dry milk powder

6 tablespoons superfine flour, such as Wondra

1 cup low-fat milk

¼ cup chopped fresh flat-leaf parsley

About ⅓ cup pecans, toasted and chopped

Heat the oil in a large pot and sauté the garlic until it's sizzling, about 1 minute. Add the squash, tomatoes, broth, dill, celery, salt, and pepper. Bring to a simmer, cover, and cook 30 minutes. Puree in batches in a food processor, or if you wish, mash the squash and tomatoes into the broth. Return the soup to a simmer.

Whisk the dry milk and flour into the liquid milk and pour into the soup, stirring constantly until the soup is bubbling and slightly thickened, about 5 minutes. Simmer for 3 minutes. Stir in the parsley. Garnish each serving with a tablespoon of chopped pecans.

Kilocalories 186 Kc • Protein 5 gm • Fat 8 gm • Percent of calories from fat 36% • Cholesterol 3 mg • Dietary fiber 2 gm • Sodium 73 mg • Calcium 101 mg

SOUPS AND CHOWDERS

Butternut and Bell Pepper Chowder

MAKES **6** SERVINGS

This is a surprisingly "creamy" yet low-fat chowder, very satisfying on a chilly fall evening.

2 tablespoons olive oil
1 red bell pepper, seeded and diced
1 green bell pepper, seeded and diced
1 jalapeño chili, seeded and minced (wear rubber gloves)
1 large yellow onion, chopped
2 cups 1-inch chunks of butternut squash, peeled (about ½ pound)
2 medium potatoes, peeled and cut into 1-inch chunks

2 cups chicken or vegetable stock (pages 10, 11) or canned low-sodium broth
3 cups low-fat milk
¼ cup nonfat dry milk powder
3 tablespoons superfine flour, such as Wondra
½ teaspoon ground cumin
¼ teaspoon salt
¼ teaspoon white pepper
2 tablespoons chopped fresh cilantro or flat-leaf parsley

Heat the oil in a large pot and sauté the peppers, chili, and onion until softened, about 5 minutes. Add the squash, potatoes, and stock. Bring to a simmer and cook, covered, until the vegetables are tender, about 15 minutes. Add 2 cups of the milk, but don't boil yet. If necessary, remove from the heat until ready to add the flour mixture.

Whisk the dry milk, flour, cumin, salt, and pepper into the remaining cup of liquid milk until blended, and pour the mixture into the soup. Cook over medium heat, stirring constantly, until bubbling and slightly thickened, about 5 minutes. Reduce the heat to very low and simmer 3 minutes longer, stirring occasionally. Stir the cilantro or parsley into the chowder before serving.

Kilocalories 304 Kc • Protein 10 gm • Fat 7 gm • Percent of calories from fat 21% • Cholesterol 10 mg • Dietary fiber 6 gm • Sodium 193 mg • Calcium 216 mg

Curried Butternut Soup with Pesto

Pretty to look at with its swirl of green, this soup makes an attractive first course for a dinner party.

2 tablespoons olive oil
1 large yellow onion, chopped
4 to 5 cups 1-inch chunks of
  butternut squash, peeled
  (about 1¼ pounds)
3 cups vegetable or chicken
  stock (pages 11, 10) or canned
  low-sodium broth

2 tablespoons low-sodium
  tomato paste
2 teaspoons mild curry powder
Freshly ground black pepper
Salt (optional)
⅓ cup Parsley Pesto (page 14)

In a large pot, heat the oil and sauté the onion until it's soft and yellow, 5 minutes. Add the squash, stock, tomato paste, curry, and pepper to taste. Bring to a boil, reduce the heat, and simmer, covered, for 30 minutes. Taste the soup to determine if you need salt.

Puree the soup in batches. Return to the pot to reheat. If it's too thick, add a little more broth. Serve the soup with a swirl of pesto in each bowl.

Kilocalories 298 Kc • Protein 6 gm • Fat 17 gm • Percent of calories from fat 49% • Cholesterol 0 mg • Dietary fiber 9 gm • Sodium 113 mg • Calcium 113 mg

Pumpkin Soup Provençal

2 tablespoons olive oil
1 medium yellow onion,
  chopped
2 garlic cloves, minced
4 cups vegetable or chicken
  stock (pages 11, 10) or canned
  low-sodium broth
4 cups 1-inch pumpkin chunks
  or butternut squash, peeled
  (1 pound)
½ teaspoon minced fresh thyme
  or ¼ teaspoon dried
½ teaspoon minced fresh sage
  or ¼ teaspoon dried leaves

¼ teaspoon salt
¼ teaspoon freshly ground black
  pepper
Dash of cayenne
Dash of ground nutmeg
2 tablespoons nonfat dry milk
  powder
2 tablespoons superfine flour,
  such as Wondra
1 cup low-fat milk
3 tablespoons chopped fresh
  flat-leaf parsley as a garnish

In a large pot, sauté the onion in the oil until it is soft and yellow, about 5 minutes. Add the garlic during the last minute. Add the stock, pumpkin, thyme, sage, salt, black pepper, cayenne, and nutmeg. Bring to a simmer and cook, covered, until the pumpkin is tender, about 20 minutes. Mash the pumpkin into the soup or puree in a food processor in batches, returning the soup to the same pan. Reheat the soup.

Whisk the dry milk and flour into the liquid milk. Add all at once to the simmering soup and stir constantly until slightly thickened, about 2 minutes. Simmer 3 minutes. Garnish with chopped parsley.

Kilocalories 130 Kc • Protein 4 gm • Fat 6 gm • Percent of calories from fat 37% • Cholesterol 3 mg • Dietary fiber 1 gm • Sodium 151 mg • Calcium 87 mg

Halloween Pumpkin and Apple Soup

———————————— ■ ————————————

MAKES **8** SERVINGS

A "sugar" pumpkin is small (2 to 4 pounds). It's a sweet variety grown especially for eating, not carving.

1 (2-pound) "sugar" pumpkin, quartered and seeded (butternut squash can be substituted)
1 tablespoon canola oil
1 medium yellow onion, diced
1 celery stalk with leaves, diced
3 Granny Smith or other tart apples, peeled and diced

5 cups chicken or vegetable stock (pages 10, 11) or canned low-sodium broth
½ teaspoon ground ginger
½ teaspoon ground allspice
¼ teaspoon ground cloves
⅛ teaspoon cayenne, or more to taste
1 tablespoon fresh lemon juice

Preheat the oven to 425 degrees F.

Arrange the pumpkin (or squash), cut side up, in a roasting pan and place it on the middle shelf. Pour in about 1 inch of water and roast the vegetable until it's tender, about 45 minutes (longer for the squash). Cool completely. Peel and roughly mash the vegetable.

In a large pot, heat the oil and sauté the onion and celery until lightly colored, 3 minutes. Add the apples, stock, ginger, allspice, cloves, and cayenne. Stir in the pumpkin. Simmer for 15 to 20 minutes, until the apples and pumpkin are very tender. Puree in batches in a food processor or blender. (Do not overfill; remember that hot foods bubble up.) Or, if you prefer, use a large whisk to partially puree the soup. Stir in the lemon juice and serve.

Kilocalories 106 Kc • Protein 3 gm • Fat 2 gm • Percent of calories from fat 20% • Cholesterol 1 mg • Dietary fiber 2 gm • Sodium 32 mg • Calcium 34 mg

Tomato, Bell Pepper, and Potato Soup

■

MAKES 6 SERVINGS

There's plenty of vitamin C in this medley of vegetables!

2 tablespoons olive oil
1 yellow onion, chopped
1 garlic clove, chopped
1 red bell pepper, seeded and
  chopped
1 (28-ounce) can imported
  Italian tomatoes with juice
1 pound potatoes, peeled
  and diced
4 cups chicken or vegetable
  stock (pages 10, 11) or canned
  low-sodium broth

½ teaspoon dried thyme
½ teaspoon dried dill
½ teaspoon dried basil
¼ teaspoon salt
Freshly ground black pepper
2 tablespoons cornstarch
1 cup low-fat milk

Heat the oil in a large pot and sauté the onion, garlic, and bell pepper until they are soft but not brown, 3 to 5 minutes. Add the tomatoes and continue cooking until the tomatoes soften a bit, 10 minutes. Add the potatoes, broth, herbs, salt, and pepper to taste, and simmer the soup until the potatoes are quite tender, about 10 minutes. Puree the soup in batches and return it to a simmer in the pot.

Mix the cornstarch with the milk until there are no lumps. Pour the milk all at once into the simmering soup, and stir constantly until it bubbles and thickens slightly, about 2 minutes. Simmer 3 minutes before serving.

Kilocalories 210 Kc • Protein 6 gm • Fat 6 gm • Percent of calories from fat 26% • Cholesterol 4 mg • Dietary fiber 4 gm • Sodium 167 mg • Calcium 109 mg

Vegetable-Cheddar Chowder

MAKES 6 SERVINGS

Especially for cheese lovers of all ages, this chowder is a tasty way to enjoy lots of antioxidant-rich vegetables in one dish.

2 tablespoons olive oil
1 large yellow onion, chopped
2 celery stalks with leaves, chopped
2 carrots, cut diagonally into ½-inch slices
1 large potato, cut into 1-inch pieces
2½ cups vegetable or chicken stock (pages 11, 10) or canned low-sodium broth
1 teaspoon chopped fresh thyme or ¼ teaspoon dried

⅛ teaspoon white pepper
A few dashes of cayenne
2 cups fresh broccoli, cut into small florets and ½-inch slices of stalk
¼ cup nonfat dry milk powder
3 tablespoons superfine flour, such as Wondra
1½ cups low-fat milk
¾ cup coarsely grated sharp Cheddar cheese

Heat the oil in a large pot and sauté the onion, celery, and carrots until they are lightly colored. Add the potato, stock, thyme, white pepper, and cayenne. Simmer until the carrot and potato are nearly tender, 8 to 10 minutes. Add the broccoli, bring to a simmer again, and continue cooking until all the vegetables are tender, about 5 minutes more.

In a saucepan, whisk the dry milk and flour into the liquid milk. Cook over medium-high heat, stirring constantly, until bubbling and thickened, about 5 minutes. Simmer over very low heat for 3 minutes, stirring often. Remove from the heat and stir in the cheese until it has melted. Whisk about 1 cup of the hot broth or more into the sauce, until it's quite thin, then stir the sauce into the soup.

Kilocalories 245 Kc • Protein 10 gm • Fat 10 gm • Percent of calories from fat 34% • Cholesterol 18 mg • Dietary fiber 4 gm • Sodium 156 mg • Calcium 228 mg

SOUPS AND CHOWDERS

71

Summer Vegetable Chowder

■

MAKES 6 SERVINGS

2 tablespoons olive oil
1 large onion, chopped
1 cup chopped celery
1 red bell pepper, seeded and
    cut into triangles
1 Anaheim chili, seeded and
    chopped
2 cups peeled seeded chopped
    tomatoes
1 pound new potatoes, peeled or
    unpeeled, cut into 1-inch
    chunks if large or halved
    if small
4 cups vegetable or chicken
    stock (pages 11, 10) or canned
    low-sodium broth

1½ cups fresh shelled peas
    or 1 (10-ounce) package
    frozen peas
1 large or 2 small summer
    squash, cut into 1-inch chunks
¼ teaspoon salt
⅛ teaspoon white pepper
¼ cup nonfat dry milk powder
3 tablespoons cornstarch
1 cup low-fat milk
2 tablespoons chopped fresh
    flat-leaf parsley
1 tablespoon chopped
    fresh basil

In a large pot, heat the oil and sauté the onion, celery, bell pepper, and Anaheim chili until they are softened, 3 to 5 minutes. Add the tomatoes, potatoes, and stock. Cover and simmer for 10 minutes. Add the peas, squash, salt, and pepper. Cover and simmer for 5 to 10 minutes. Test that all the vegetables are tender; simmer longer if necessary.

Whisk the dry milk and cornstarch into the liquid milk, and add it to the simmering chowder. Stir constantly until the mixture bubbles and thickens slightly, about 2 minutes. Stir in the parsley and basil.

Kilocalories 238 Kc • Protein 8 gm • Fat 6 gm • Percent of calories from fat 22% • Cholesterol 3 mg • Dietary fiber 6 gm • Sodium 185 mg • Calcium 106 mg

Winter Root Vegetable Soup with Fresh Dill

———————————— ■ ————————————

This satisfying "creamy" soup with very little fat is just the dish for a cold winter day.

2 tablespoons olive oil
1 large yellow onion, chopped
2 medium carrots, sliced
2 red potatoes, peeled and diced
½ pound parsnips, pared and sliced
2 garlic cloves, chopped

4 cups vegetable or chicken stock (pages 11, 10) or canned low-sodium broth
Salt (optional)
Freshly ground black pepper
1 tablespoon chopped fresh dill

Heat the oil in a large pot and sauté the onion, carrots, potatoes, parsnips, and garlic until they begin to change color but are not browned, 5 minutes. Add the stock, bring to a boil, and simmer, covered, until all the vegetables are quite tender, about 20 minutes. Scoop out the solids with a slotted spoon and puree them in a food processor. Through the feed tube, add about 1 cup of the liquid to make a smooth mixture. Return the vegetables to the pot and whisk until smoothly blended. Taste the soup to determine if you need salt. Add pepper to taste. Stir in the dill.

Kilocalories 252 Kc • Protein 5 gm • Fat 8 gm • Percent of calories from fat 26% • Cholesterol 0 mg • Dietary fiber 6 gm • Sodium 67 mg • Calcium 49 mg

Barley and Vegetable Soup

Dishes rich in antioxidants are often rich in fiber as well, like this barley-thickened soup.

½ cup barley
8 cups chicken or vegetable
   stock (pages 10, 11) or canned
   low-sodium broth
2 tablespoons olive oil
1 large yellow onion, chopped
5 ounces thinly sliced
   mushrooms
1 cup diced carrots
1 cup diced celery

1 cup peeled seeded chopped
   tomatoes
1 small zucchini, diced
1 tablespoon *each* chopped
   fresh basil and cilantro or
   ½ teaspoon dried
¼ teaspoon salt
Freshly ground black pepper
   to taste

In a saucepan, combine the barley with 3 cups of the broth, bring the mixture to a boil, and simmer over low heat, covered, until the barley is tender, about 45 minutes.

In a large pot, heat the oil and sauté the onion and mushrooms until lightly colored, about 5 minutes. Add the remaining 5 cups broth, the vegetables, herbs, and seasonings, and cook until the vegetables are tender, about 15 minutes. Add the barley and its liquid, if not absorbed, and continue to cook for 5 minutes or so to blend the flavors.

Kilocalories 139 Kc • Protein 6 gm • Fat 4 gm • Percent of calories from fat 31% • Cholesterol 2 mg • Dietary fiber 4 gm • Sodium 138 mg • Calcium 23 mg

BARLEY AND ARTICHOKE SOUP: Follow the preceding recipe, substituting 8 to 10 artichoke hearts—fresh (well trimmed), frozen, or canned—halved or quartered, depending on size, for the zucchini.

Kilocalories 158 Kc • Protein 7 gm • Fat 4 gm • Percent of calories from fat 26% • Cholesterol 2 mg • Dietary fiber 6 gm • Sodium 178 mg • Calcium 40 mg

Salmon, Corn, and Zucchini Chowder

■

MAKES 6 SERVINGS

A trio of summer favorites teams up in this delicious soup. It can easily be the main dish—just add Tossed Greens with Tomato and Cucumber (page 291).

2 tablespoons olive oil
1 red bell pepper, seeded
  and diced
1 large yellow onion, chopped
2 medium potatoes, cut into
  1-inch chunks
1 medium zucchini, cut into
  1-inch chunks
2 cups vegetable stock (page 11)
  or canned low-sodium broth
1 cup fresh or frozen corn
  kernels

1¼ pounds skinless salmon
  fillet, cut into 1-inch pieces
3 cups low-fat milk
¼ cup nonfat dry milk powder
3 tablespoons superfine flour,
  such as Wondra
¼ teaspoon salt
¼ teaspoon white pepper
2 tablespoons chopped fresh
  cilantro or flat-leaf parsley

Heat the oil in a large pot and sauté the bell pepper and onion until softened, about 5 minutes. Add the potatoes, zucchini, and stock. Bring to a simmer and cook, covered, until the vegetables are tender, about 15 minutes. Add the corn and salmon, and simmer 3 minutes longer. Remove from the heat. Add 2 cups of the milk.

Whisk the dry milk, flour, salt, and pepper into the remaining 1 cup liquid milk until blended, and pour the mixture into the soup. Cook over medium heat, stirring constantly, until bubbling and slightly thickened, about 5 minutes. Reduce the heat to very low and simmer 3 minutes longer, or until the salmon is cooked through, stirring occasionally. Stir the cilantro or parsley into the chowder before serving.

Kilocalories 367 Kc • Protein 27 gm • Fat 13 gm • Percent of calories from fat 32% • Cholesterol 61 mg • Dietary fiber 3 gm • Sodium 227 mg • Calcium 190 mg

Oyster and Vegetable Stew, Mexican Style

MAKES 4 SERVINGS

Oysters are a major source of zinc, the "unsung antioxidant."

1 pint shucked oysters
2 tablespoons canola oil
1 green bell pepper, seeded
   and diced
1 Anaheim chili, seeded and
   chopped
1 jalapeño chili, seeded and
   minced (wear rubber gloves)
1 large yellow onion, chopped

1 garlic clove, finely chopped
1 (8-ounce) bottle clam juice
1 (1-pound) can low-sodium
   chopped tomatoes with juice
2 cups peeled diced potatoes
2 tablespoons drained capers
½ teaspoon hot pepper sauce
⅛ teaspoon pepper, or more
   to taste

Drain the oysters, reserving their liquor. Cut any extra large oysters in half.

In a large pot, heat the oil and slowly "sweat" the bell pepper, chilies, onion, and garlic until soft but not brown, about 10 minutes. Add the oyster liquor, clam juice, tomatoes, potatoes, capers, hot pepper sauce, and pepper. Cover and simmer until the potatoes are tender, 10 to 15 minutes. Add the oysters and simmer 5 minutes longer.

Kilocalories 288 Kc • Protein 13 gm • Fat 11 gm • Percent of calories from fat 32% • Cholesterol 66 mg • Dietary fiber 4 gm • Sodium 581 mg • Calcium 88 mg

ANTIOXIDANT POWER

76

Chilled Peach and Lime Soup

———————◼———————

Here's a nice and easy July pick-me-up.

3 cups peeled fresh peach slices
(about 4 large very ripe
peaches)
1 cup or more orange juice
2 tablespoons lime juice (1 lime)

1 (8-ounce) container nonfat
peach or vanilla yogurt
4 thin slices unpeeled lime for
garnish

In a food processor or blender, puree the peaches with the orange juice
and lime juice. Chill. Just before serving, whisk in the yogurt. Serve in glass
bowls or stemmed water glasses. Garnish each serving with a lime slice.

Kilocalories 117 Kc • Protein 5 gm • Fat 0 gm • Percent of calories from fat
2% • Cholesterol 0 mg • Dietary fiber 3 gm • Sodium 43 mg • Calcium 126 mg

Iced Strawberry Soup

---■---

This can be a starter or dessert—it's all up to you!

1 quart fresh strawberries
1½ cups orange juice
2 tablespoons sugar

1 (8-ounce) container nonfat
strawberry or vanilla yogurt

Wash and hull the strawberries, reserving 4 small whole berries. In a food processor or blender, puree the remaining berries with the orange juice and sugar. Chill. Just before serving, whisk in the yogurt. Serve in glass bowls or stemmed water glasses. Slice the whole berries and float them on top for a garnish.

Kilocalories 226 Kc • Protein 5 gm • Fat 0 gm • Percent of calories from fat 1% • Cholesterol 0 mg • Dietary fiber 4 gm • Sodium 42 mg • Calcium 111 mg

ANTIOXIDANT POWER

Grains, Rice, and Pasta

With their wonderful variety, grains, rice, and pasta offer many pleasing and popular ways to add antioxidant-rich foods to our meals. Whenever possible, choosing unrefined grains, such as brown rice and whole wheat pasta, adds even more antioxidant power to a dish because whole grains are a good source of vitamin E. But even refined grains, when combined with antioxidant vegetables, can create a nutritious as well as delicious dish.

Cooking pasta is so easy, it qualifies as a genuine "fast food," but there are a few important rules. Four to five quarts of water are needed for one pound of pasta and at least three quarts for a half pound. If you are adding salt, do so when the water is boiling, just before adding the pasta, 2 teaspoons per pound. Don't worry—most of that will be drained away. Taste is the best test for perfect pasta—the cooking time given in the package directions should be considered a guide only. If the pasta will be subjected to further cooking, as would be the case with a soup or casserole, it's best to undercook it a bit. And pasta must be sauced immediately after draining so that it won't stick together. It should be served promptly, too, to prevent its getting mushy while being kept warm in the serving dish.

A pasta dish can be a first course, a main dish, or a side dish—however the cook wishes to present it. A protein-rich dish such as Chicken Primavera with Shells or Tofu and Broccoli with Shells would make a substantial main dish, whereas Basil Asparagus with Linguine could be a light starter or side dish. It's all up to you and the menu you have planned.

Methods of cooking the grain foods vary considerably, so specific recipe directions must apply. But there is one general rule: Whether you're cooking rice, bulgur, or couscous, the grains should not be allowed to clump together. Fluff them up with a fork to separate them very well before serving.

Polenta, an Italian cornmeal dish flavored with cheese, is also included in this chapter. It can be served hot, spooned out like mashed potatoes, or chilled, cut into attractive squares, and baked or fried to reheat. Either way, it makes a marvelous background for spicy and succulent vegetable toppings.

Risotto with Radicchio and Pinto Beans

It's "red beans and rice," Venetian style.

1 tablespoon olive oil
1 yellow onion, chopped
1½ cups arborio rice
About 4 cups chicken or
vegetable stock (pages 10, 11)
or canned low-sodium broth

1 cup shredded radicchio
1 cup canned low-sodium pinto
beans, drained and rinsed
⅓ cup freshly grated Parmesan
cheese
Freshly ground black pepper

Heat the oil in a large heavy saucepan, and sauté the onion until limp and yellowed, 3 to 5 minutes. Add the rice and cook, stirring, until all the grains are coated with oil. Meanwhile, have the broth simmering in another saucepan. Add 1 cup of the broth to the rice and simmer, stirring often, until it's almost all absorbed. Add 1 cup of the broth and the radicchio. Continue cooking and adding broth, with frequent stirring, until the rice is tender and the mixture is creamy. You may not need all the broth. Total cooking time: 20 to 25 minutes. Stir in the beans and cook 1 minute longer.

Remove from the heat and stir in the cheese. Add pepper to taste. Serve immediately.

Kilocalories 270 Kc • Protein 8 gm • Fat 4 gm • Percent of calories from fat 15% • Cholesterol 4 mg • Dietary fiber 3 gm • Sodium 106 mg • Calcium 73 mg

GRAINS, RICE, AND PASTA

Oven-baked Brown Rice Pilaf
with Bell Peppers

■

The finished pilaf can be topped with grated Parmesan cheese, or a bowl of nonfat plain yogurt can be passed at the table.

2 tablespoons olive oil
1 medium yellow onion, chopped
1 red bell pepper, diced
1 green bell pepper, diced
1 garlic clove, minced
1 cup brown rice (not instant)

3 cups vegetable or chicken stock (pages 11, 10) or canned low-sodium broth
Freshly ground black pepper
1 tablespoon minced fresh flat-leaf parsley

Preheat the oven to 375 degrees F.

In a Dutch oven or other heavy range-to-oven pan, heat the oil and sauté the onion and bell peppers until they are sizzling and fragrant, 3 minutes. Add the garlic and cook 1 minute longer. Add the rice and stir over low heat to coat each grain with the oil.

Add the stock and bring to a boil. Add pepper to taste. Cover and place the casserole, with broth boiling, into the oven. Bake on the middle shelf until all the liquid is absorbed and the rice tender, about 50 minutes. Fluff well. Stir in the parsley before serving.

Kilocalories 288 Kc • Protein 5 gm • Fat 9 gm • Percent of calories from fat 26% • Cholesterol 0 mg • Dietary fiber 3 gm • Sodium 36 mg • Calcium 30 mg

Oven-baked Bulgur Pilaf with Carrots

This nutty-flavored staple of the Middle East is an excellent source of whole grain goodness. Serve it as a side dish with fish or chicken.

2 tablespoons olive oil
½ cup sliced scallions
1 small green bell pepper, seeded and diced
2 cups coarsely grated carrots
2 cups vegetable or chicken stock (pages 11, 10) or canned low-sodium broth

⅛ teaspoon freshly ground black pepper
1 cup bulgur (cracked wheat)
1 tablespoon minced fresh cilantro

Preheat the oven to 350 degrees F.

In a Dutch oven or other heavy range-to-oven casserole with a cover, heat the oil and sauté the scallions, bell pepper, and carrots until lightly colored, about 10 minutes. Add the stock and pepper, and bring it to a boil. Add the bulgur, cover, and reduce the heat. Place the covered, simmering casserole in the oven and bake until all the liquid is absorbed and the carrots are tender, about 20 minutes. Remove the cover and stir in the cilantro. Fluff well before serving.

Kilocalories 232 Kc • Protein 6 gm • Fat 8 gm • Percent of calories from fat 28% • Cholesterol 0 mg • Dietary fiber 9 gm • Sodium 49 mg • Calcium 39 mg

GRAINS, RICE, AND PASTA

Whole Wheat Couscous with Apricots and Pistachios

Couscous is North African pasta. Its grains are as small as pastina and even more delicate. The directions in this recipe are for whole wheat couscous, found in natural food stores; cooking is best done in a double boiler. If you substitute the white couscous found in supermarkets, follow the general package directions, no double boiler needed, adding the ingredients indicated below. This couscous dish is a perfect companion to roasted chicken or turkey

2 cups vegetable or chicken
   stock (pages 11, 10) or canned
   low-sodium broth
¼ teaspoon ground cardamom
¼ teaspoon ground cumin

⅛ teaspoon ground cinnamon
¼ cup chopped dried apricots
¼ cup dried currants
1 cup whole wheat couscous
¼ cup shelled pistachio nuts

Bring the stock to a boil in the top of a double boiler. Whisk in the cardamom, cumin, and cinnamon. Stir in the apricots and currants. Gradually add the couscous. Stir until the mixture boils again. Place it over 1 inch of simmering water, cover, and cook 15 minutes. Uncover and fluff well. Stir in the nuts. Spoon the couscous onto a medium serving platter, breaking up any remaining clumps.

Kilocalories 304 Kc • Protein 10 gm • Fat 6 gm • Percent of calories from fat 15% • Cholesterol 0 mg • Dietary fiber 9 gm • Sodium 23 mg • Calcium 35 mg

Quinoa with Roasted Sweet Potatoes

MAKES 4 SERVINGS

Quinoa (pronounced keen-*wah) was a staple of the Inca empire. Recently rediscovered as a protein-packed healthy grain food, quinoa must always be rinsed before cooking to remove any residue of a natural bitter coating.*

1 large sweet potato, peeled and cut into 1-inch pieces (¾ pound)
1 medium yellow onion, peeled and diced

1 cup diced fennel or celery
2 tablespoons olive oil
½ teaspoon salt
¾ cup quinoa

Preheat the oven to 375 degrees F.

Toss the potato, onion, and fennel with the oil and ¼ teaspoon salt. Arrange the vegetables in a large gratin dish from which you can serve and bake until they are tender, turning them once during the cooking time— 35 to 40 minutes.

Meanwhile, thoroughly rinse the quinoa in a strainer. Put it into a medium saucepan with 1½ cups water and the remaining ¼ teaspoon salt. Bring to a boil, reduce the heat, and simmer, covered, until all the water is absorbed, 12 to 15 minutes. When quinoa is cooked, the grains turn from white to transparent and the spiral-like germ unfurls from the grain.

Gently mix the quinoa with the roasted vegetables and serve.

Kilocalories 288 Kc • Protein 6 gm • Fat 9 gm • Percent of calories from fat 26% • Cholesterol 0 mg • Dietary fiber 6 gm • Sodium 176 mg • Calcium 63 mg

GRAINS, RICE, AND PASTA

85

Braised Fennel with Polenta

Almost any vegetable sauce can make a delicious topping for polenta—Italy's answer to our "cornmeal mush."

About 3½ cups polenta
  (page 12)
2 tablespoons olive oil
2 fennel bulbs, cored and cut
  into wedges
1 garlic clove, chopped
1 cup tomato sauce (page 14
  or use store-bought sauce
  from a jar)

1 tablespoon chopped fresh
  basil or ½ teaspoon dried
½ teaspoon chopped fresh
  rosemary or a pinch of dried

Start preparing the polenta, which takes 45 minutes to cook.

In a Dutch oven, heat the oil and sauté the fennel until it begins to brown, 8 to 10 minutes. Add the garlic and cook 1 minute longer. Add the tomato sauce and ¼ cup water. Cover the pan and cook over very low heat, stirring occasionally, until the fennel is quite tender, 15 to 20 minutes. Stir in the herbs during the last 5 minutes.

Spread the polenta on a platter and top with the fennel.

Kilocalories 289 Kc • Protein 10 gm • Fat 11 gm • Percent of calories from fat 34% • Cholesterol 9 mg • Dietary fiber 5 gm • Sodium 252 mg • Calcium 176 mg

ANTIOXIDANT POWER

86

Broiled Eggplant with Pesto on Polenta

MAKES 4 SERVINGS

Since eggplant acts as a sponge for oil, it's best to broil rather than fry it whenever possible.

1 large eggplant (1 to
  1¼ pounds)
Salt
About 3 cups polenta (page 12)
1 garlic clove, sliced

2 tablespoons olive oil, or more
  if needed
About ½ cup Basil Pesto
  (page 13)

Peel, slice, and salt the eggplant. Allow the slices to drain in a colander for a half hour.

Make the polenta and keep it warm. Meanwhile, combine the garlic and oil, and allow it to marinate.

Preheat the broiler. Rinse and press the eggplant slices dry between paper towels. Discard the garlic and brush the slices on both sides with the oil. Broil them until they are lightly colored and tender, about 5 minutes per side. Spread the slices with pesto.

Spread the hot polenta on a platter. Top with the eggplant.

EGGPLANT AND POLENTA WITH TOMATO SAUCE: Follow the preceding recipe, omitting the pesto. Arrange the eggplant slices on the platter of polenta and ladle about 1½ cups Tomato-Mushroom Sauce (page 15) over all.

Kilocalories 372 Kc • Protein 11 gm • Fat 22 gm • Percent of calories from fat 53% • Cholesterol 7 mg • Dietary fiber 6 gm • Sodium 257 mg • Calcium 146 mg

Swiss Chard, Garlic, and Anchovies with Polenta

MAKES **4** SERVINGS

Swiss chard's red stalks are a reminder that this vegetable is a relative of the beet family.

1 bunch Swiss chard (about ¾ pound)

2 tablespoons extra-virgin olive oil

1 red bell pepper, seeded and cut into strips

2 garlic cloves, finely chopped

4 anchovy fillets, rinsed in wine vinegar

About ⅛ teaspoon freshly ground black pepper

About ⅛ teaspoon hot red pepper flakes

3½ cups hot cooked polenta (page 12)

½ cup finely slivered Asiago cheese

Wash the chard well. Coarsely chop the leaves and tender stems. Cut larger stalks into 2-inch pieces.

In a 12-inch skillet, heat the oil and sauté the bell pepper, garlic, and anchovies over very low heat until the garlic is softened, 3 minutes. The anchovies should be soft enough to break up with the back of a spoon. Stir in the black and hot red peppers. Add the chard and ¼ cup water. Cover and simmer until the greens and stalks are tender, 6 to 8 minutes.

Spoon freshly cooked polenta onto a large platter. Top with the greens and pan juices. Sprinkle with cheese and serve.

Kilocalories 329 Kc • Protein 16 gm • Fat 14 gm • Percent of calories from fat 39% • Cholesterol 20 mg • Dietary fiber 4 gm • Sodium 691 mg • Calcium 337 mg

MUSTARD GREENS WITH POLENTA: Follow the preceding recipe, substituting mustard greens for the chard. Trim off and discard tough stems. Coarsely chop the leaves.

Kilocalories 341 Kc • Protein 16 gm • Fat 14 gm • Percent of calories from fat 39% • Cholesterol 20 mg • Dietary fiber 5 gm • Sodium 526 mg • Calcium 384 mg

Fresh Garden Sauce with Polenta

■

MAKES 4 SERVINGS

Made from local early summer produce, this dish might also be called Polenta Primavera.

2 tablespoons olive oil
1 cup chopped scallions
1 Italian frying pepper, diced
1 garlic clove, minced
2 cups peeled seeded chopped fresh ripe tomatoes
¼ teaspoon salt
Freshly ground black pepper
1 medium zucchini, thinly sliced
1 large carrot, thinly sliced

½ pound fresh young green beans, ends trimmed
1 tablespoon minced fresh flat-leaf parsley
1 teaspoon minced fresh basil
1 teaspoon minced fresh marjoram
3½ cups hot cooked polenta (page 12)
Freshly grated Parmesan cheese

Heat the oil in a large skillet and sauté the scallions and pepper until they are softened, 3 to 5 minutes. Add the garlic and cook 1 minute longer. Add the tomatoes, salt, and pepper to taste, and sauté, stirring often, for 5 minutes. Add the zucchini, carrot, and green beans. Cover and simmer until the vegetables are tender, 5 to 7 minutes. Stir in the herbs.

Spoon freshly cooked polenta onto a large platter. Top with the garden sauce. Pass grated cheese at the table.

Kilocalories 319 Kc • Protein 12 gm • Fat 11 gm • Percent of calories from fat 31% • Cholesterol 9 mg • Dietary fiber 8 gm • Sodium 380 mg • Calcium 210 mg

Basil Asparagus with Linguine

■

With the asparagus spears left whole, this is a somewhat messy-to-eat but beautiful and delectable spring pasta dish.

1 pound fresh asparagus
2 tablespoons olive oil
2 garlic cloves, minced
1 (1-pound) can Italian-style
  plum tomatoes in puree (not
  ground tomatoes)

¼ teaspoon salt
Freshly ground black pepper
1 tablespoon fresh basil, minced
12 ounces linguine
Freshly grated Parmesan cheese

Trim off the woody ends of the asparagus. Put 1 cup water in a large skillet, add the asparagus, and bring to a boil. Cover and simmer over low heat until the asparagus is just tender, 3 to 5 minutes. Drain from the pan; using the pan cover to hold back the vegetable is the easiest way. Remove the asparagus and dry the pan.

In the same skillet, heat the oil and sauté the garlic for 1 minute. Add the tomatoes, breaking them up with a fork. Add salt and pepper to taste, and simmer the sauce, uncovered, for about 20 minutes, until slightly thickened. Stir in the basil. Add the asparagus.

Meanwhile, cook the linguine according to package directions. Drain and spoon into a large shallow serving dish. Top with the asparagus and sauce, stirring around the edges to let the sauce penetrate the pasta. Pass grated cheese at the table.

Kilocalories 435 Kc • Protein 14 gm • Fat 8 gm • Percent of calories from fat 17% • Cholesterol 0 mg • Dietary fiber 6 gm • Sodium 169 mg • Calcium 81 mg

Broccoli with Tomato Sauce and Rigatoni

MAKES 4 SIDE-DISH SERVINGS, 2 MAIN-DISH SERVINGS

Here's a powerhouse of antioxidants in one dish!

2 broccoli crowns (¾ to
  1 pound)
¾ cup chicken or vegetable
  stock (pages 10, 11) or canned
  low-sodium broth
1 cup tomato sauce (page 14
  or use store-bought sauce
  from a jar)

Hot red pepper flakes
6 to 7 ounces rigatoni
Freshly grated Parmesan cheese

Cut the broccoli into thin (about ½-inch) stalks with florets attached. Put them into a 10-inch skillet with the stock, bring to a simmer, cover, and cook until the broccoli is just tender, about 5 minutes. Stir in the tomato sauce. Season with hot pepper flakes to taste.

Meanwhile, cook the rigatoni according to package directions. Stir the rigatoni into the broccoli, then transfer to a serving dish. Pass grated cheese at the table.

Kilocalories 231 Kc • Protein 9 gm • Fat 4 gm • Percent of calories from fat 16% • Cholesterol 0 mg • Dietary fiber 4 gm • Sodium 91 mg • Calcium 62 mg

Tofu and Broccoli with Shells

■

Carrot Slaw with Scallions (page 319) would make a complementary accompaniment to this pasta dish.

1 pound broccoli crowns
2 tablespoons olive oil, or more if needed
1 (14-ounce) package firm tofu, diced, well drained
2 garlic cloves, minced
1 (28-ounce) can Italian plum tomatoes in puree, chopped into 1-inch pieces
½ cup dry white wine
¼ teaspoon salt
¼ teaspoon freshly ground black pepper
1 tablespoon chopped fresh basil or 1 teaspoon dried
2 tablespoons chopped fresh flat-leaf parsley
12 ounces medium shell pasta
Freshly grated Parmesan cheese

Chop the broccoli into small florets and 1-inch slices of stalk.

Heat the oil in a large skillet. Stir-fry the tofu until it's lightly browned on all sides, about 5 minutes. Remove the tofu with a slotted spoon and reserve it.

Add more oil if needed and sauté the garlic for 1 minute. Add the tomatoes, wine, salt, and pepper to the skillet, and simmer, uncovered, stirring often, for 15 minutes. Add the broccoli, tofu, basil, and parsley, cover, and continue to simmer, stirring once or twice, for 5 minutes, or until the broccoli is tender-crisp.

Meanwhile, cook the shells according to package directions and drain them. Spoon the pasta into a serving dish and toss with the tofu-broccoli sauce. Pass the cheese at the table.

Kilocalories 574 Kc • Protein 26 gm • Fat 12 gm • Percent of calories from fat 20% • Cholesterol 0 mg • Dietary fiber 9 gm • Sodium 220 mg • Calcium 309 mg

Broccoli de Rabe and Mushrooms with Vermicelli

■

This is hearty enough to be a vegetarian main dish. Cannellini, Bell Pepper, and Tomato Salad (page 309) makes a colorful, compatible side dish.

1 large bunch broccoli de rabe
  (¾ to 1 pound)
2½ tablespoons olive oil
10 ounces white or brown
  mushrooms, cleaned and
  sliced

3 large garlic cloves, minced
1 cup vegetable or chicken stock
  (pages 11, 10) or canned low-
  sodium broth
Hot red pepper flakes
12 ounces vermicelli

Wash the broccoli de rabe well, trim off the tough stems, and coarsely chop the bunch. Heat 2 tablespoons of the oil in a large skillet and sauté the mushrooms over high heat, stirring often. Cook until their liquid content evaporates and they begin to turn color. Lower the heat and continue to cook until they are golden brown. Remove the mushrooms with a slotted spoon.

Add the remaining ½ tablespoon of oil and sauté the garlic until it's sizzling. Add the broccoli de rabe and broth. Cover and simmer until the broccoli de rabe is tender, 7 to 10 minutes. Add the mushrooms and reheat if necessary. Season the broccoli de rabe with hot red pepper flakes to taste.

Cook the vermicelli according to package directions and drain. Transfer the pasta to a serving dish and toss with the broccoli de rabe, mushrooms, and broth.

Kilocalories 457 Kc • Protein 15 gm • Fat 10 gm • Percent of calories from fat 20% • Cholesterol 0 mg • Dietary fiber 3 gm • Sodium 36 mg • Calcium 175 mg

GRAINS, RICE, AND PASTA

Chili Bean Sauce with Fettuccine

This pasta dish is a zesty "go-along" with burgers or meat loaf.

2 tablespoons olive oil
1 medium yellow onion,
 chopped
1 green bell pepper, seeded
 and diced
1 to 2 fresh or canned jalapeño
 chilies, seeded and minced
 (wear rubber gloves)
1 garlic clove, minced
2 cups peeled seeded chopped
 fresh tomatoes or 1 (1-pound)
 can chopped tomatoes,
 undrained
1 tablespoon chopped fresh
 oregano or ½ teaspoon dried

1 teaspoon chili powder
¼ teaspoon salt
¼ teaspoon freshly ground black
 pepper
1 (15- to 16-ounce) can low-
 sodium red kidney beans,
 drained and rinsed
2 tablespoons chopped fresh
 cilantro or fresh flat-leaf
 parsley
12 ounces fettuccine
½ cup shredded Monterey Jack
 cheese

Heat the oil in a 10-inch skillet, and sauté the onion and bell pepper until softened, 5 minutes. Add the chilies and garlic, and cook 1 minute longer. Add the tomatoes, oregano, chili powder, salt, and pepper. Simmer, uncovered, stirring occasionally, for 10 minutes. Add the beans and cilantro; cook 5 minutes longer.

Meanwhile, cook the fettucine according to package directions and drain. Spoon the fettucine into a large serving dish and toss it with a little of the tomato sauce from the beans. Pour the rest of the bean sauce on top and sprinkle with the cheese.

Kilocalories 543 Kc • Protein 24 gm • Fat 10 gm • Percent of calories from fat 17% • Cholesterol 5 mg • Dietary fiber 9 gm • Sodium 217 mg • Calcium 196 mg

ANTIOXIDANT POWER

Stir-fried Sesame Cabbage with Asian Noodles

---■---

MAKES 4 SIDE-DISH SERVINGS

This easy, light pasta dish could be served with baked fish.

1 tablespoon sesame seeds
1 tablespoon canola oil
1 teaspoon sesame oil
1 bunch scallions, cut into ½-inch lengths
1 green bell pepper, seeded and cut into thin strips

2 slices fresh ginger, minced
6 cups loosely packed, thinly sliced cabbage
8 ounces thin Asian noodles or angel hair pasta
Naturally brewed reduced-sodium soy sauce

In a small pan or skillet, toast the sesame seeds over very low heat until they are golden but not brown, about 1 minute. Stir them constantly and watch carefully. As soon as they are the right color, remove them from the pan to a dish and reserve.

In a large wok or skillet, heat the oils and stir-fry the scallions, bell pepper, and ginger for 2 minutes. Add the cabbage and continue stir-frying until it's wilted and tender-crisp, about 5 minutes.

Cook the noodles according to package directions and drain them. Transfer the noodles to a serving dish and toss with the cabbage mixture. Sprinkle with sesame seeds and serve. Pass the soy sauce at the table.

Kilocalories 170 Kc • Protein 4 gm • Fat 6 gm • Percent of calories from fat 31% • Cholesterol 0 mg • Dietary fiber 3 gm • Sodium 25 mg • Calcium 89 mg

Sautéed Savoy Cabbage with Gemellini and Gorgonzola

Fresh sage is so different from dried and so special, it's worthwhile growing a pot of it on a sunny windowsill all year.

2 tablespoons olive oil
4 cups shredded savoy cabbage
  (about ½ medium head)
2 garlic cloves, minced
6 fresh sage leaves, chopped
½ cup chicken stock (page 10)
  or canned low-sodium broth

Freshly ground black pepper
8 ounces gemellini (little twists)
2 ounces crumbled Gorgonzola
  cheese

Heat the oil in a 12-inch skillet and sauté the cabbage, stirring often, until it's just tender, 3 to 5 minutes. Add the garlic and sage during the last minute. Add the broth and remove from the heat. Add pepper to taste. Reheat when the pasta is ready.

Cook the gemellini according to package directions and drain. Toss the hot pasta with the cabbage and Gorgonzola. Serve immediately.

Kilocalories 347 Kc • Protein 12 gm • Fat 12 gm • Percent of calories from fat 31% • Cholesterol 10 mg • Dietary fiber 4 gm • Sodium 222 mg • Calcium 121 mg

Cauliflower and Cranberry Beans with Orrechiette

MAKES 4 SERVINGS

Fresh cranberry beans are a joy worth the effort of shelling, but their season is short. Canned low-sodium shell beans can be substituted when fresh beans are not available.

½ large head cauliflower (4 to 5 cups small florets)

1½ pounds fresh cranberry beans, shelled (about 2 cups)

2 tablespoons olive oil

2 or 3 garlic cloves, minced

1 cup chicken stock (page 10) or canned low-sodium broth

½ teaspoon dried summer savory or dried marjoram

¼ teaspoon salt

Freshly ground black pepper

1 tablespoon chopped fresh basil

1 tablespoon chopped fresh parsley

12 ounces orrechiette (ear-shaped pasta)

Freshly grated Romano cheese

Trim, core, and separate the cauliflower into florets. Cook the florets in boiling salted water until tender-crisp, about 3 minutes. Scoop out the florets with a slotted spoon. Cook the beans in the same water until tender, 15 to 25 minutes, depending on their size. Drain the beans.

Heat the olive oil in a 12-inch skillet and sauté the garlic until it's sizzling and fragrant, about 1 minute. Add the vegetables, broth, savory, salt, and pepper to taste, and simmer the mixture for 3 minutes. Stir in the basil and parsley.

Cook the orrechiette according to package directions and drain. In a large serving dish, toss the pasta, vegetables, and ½ cup cheese. Pass more cheese at the table.

Kilocalories 571 Kc • Protein 25 gm • Fat 12 gm • Percent of calories from fat 18% • Cholesterol 11 mg • Dietary fiber 14 gm • Sodium 313 mg • Calcium 196 mg

Savory Baked Eggplant with Ziti

MAKES 2 GENEROUS SERVINGS

Sicilian green olives give this casserole a piquant flavor.

1 medium eggplant (about
  1 pound)
Salt
Olive oil
Dried oregano
Dried rosemary
1 garlic clove, minced
1½ cups peeled seeded chopped
  ripe tomatoes

⅓ cup pitted chopped Sicilian
  green olives
1 tablespoon balsamic vinegar
Freshly ground black pepper
2 tablespoons chopped fresh
  flat-leaf parsley
8 ounces ziti with lines

Peel and slice the eggplant. Salt the slices and drain them in a colander for a half hour or so. Rinse the slices and pat them dry between paper towels, pressing out excess moisture.

Preheat the oven to 350 degrees F. Brush the slices on both sides with oil and arrange them on a baking sheet. Sprinkle with dried herbs to taste. Bake in the middle of the oven until tender but not mushy, 10 to 15 minutes.

Heat 1 tablespoon oil in a large skillet and sauté the garlic until it sizzles, about 1 minute. Add the tomatoes, olives, vinegar, ⅛ teaspoon salt, and pepper to taste, and simmer the sauce, uncovered, stirring often, for 10 minutes. Cut the eggplant slices into quarters and add them to the sauce. Simmer 2 minutes. Stir in the parsley and remove from the heat.

Cook the ziti according to package directions and drain. Spoon the ziti into a large serving dish and toss with the eggplant sauce.

Kilocalories 610 Kc • Protein 18 gm • Fat 12 gm • Percent of calories from fat 18% • Cholesterol 0 mg • Dietary fiber 10 gm • Sodium 506 mg • Calcium 52 mg

Roasted Eggplant and Butternut with Penne

This dish makes an especially attractive presentation.

1 large eggplant (about
  1¼ pounds)
Salt
¾ pound butternut squash, cut
  into ½-inch pieces (about
  2½ cups)
1 red bell pepper, seeded and
  cut into strips
1 green bell pepper, seeded and
  cut into strips
6 plum tomatoes, quartered
  lengthwise, seeded
¼ cup olive oil

3 large garlic cloves, minced
1 tablespoon chopped fresh
  basil or ½ teaspoon dried
1 tablespoon chopped fresh flat-
  leaf parsley
Freshly ground black pepper
1 pound penne or ziti
½ cup vegetable or chicken
  stock (pages 11, 10) or canned
  low-sodium broth
Freshly grated Parmesan cheese
Hot red pepper flakes (optional)

Peel, slice, and salt the eggplant. Allow the slices to drain in a colander for a half hour. Rinse the slices and press them dry between paper towels. Cut them into quarters.

Preheat the oven to 400 degrees F.

Combine the eggplant, squash, bell peppers, and tomatoes in a large roasting pan that will fit them in one close layer. Toss with the olive oil. Roast on the middle shelf, turning once or twice during the cooking time, until the vegetables are tender and lightly colored, about 45 minutes. Stir in the garlic and continue cooking for 5 minutes. Remove from the oven. Sprinkle with basil, parsley, ¼ teaspoon salt, and pepper to taste.

Cook the penne according to package directions and drain. Toss the penne with the broth, roasted vegetables, and ¼ cup cheese. Pass extra cheese and hot red pepper flakes, if you wish, at the table.

Kilocalories 448 Kc • Protein 13 gm • Fat 12 gm • Percent of calories from fat 23% • Cholesterol 3 mg • Dietary fiber 7 gm • Sodium 183 mg • Calcium 108 mg

Roasted Fennel and Tomatoes with Linguine

■

MAKES 4 SERVINGS

Roasting brings out a unique flavor in tomatoes. Arranging the vegetables in one crowded layer is best because it allows them to roast while generating a little steam to tenderize them faster.

2 medium fennel bulbs
4 tablespoons olive oil
8 large ripe plum tomatoes, halved and seeded
4 garlic cloves, minced
½ cup pitted black olives
1 teaspoon chopped fresh rosemary or ¼ teaspoon dried
Salt and freshly ground black pepper

12 ounces fresh or dried linguine (fresh is particularly nice in this dish)
½ cup chicken or vegetable stock (pages 10, 11), or canned low-sodium broth, warmed
Freshly grated Parmesan cheese

Preheat the oven to 425 degrees F.

Trim and cut the fennel bulbs in half. Core the bulbs. Put aside the tougher outer covering (which is cupped around the bulb) for salad or soup and slice the inner bulbs into thin wedges. Coat a large baking pan with 1 tablespoon oil. Arrange the fennel and tomatoes in a roasting pan that just fits them. Scatter the garlic, olives, and rosemary on top. Drizzle the remaining 3 tablespoons olive oil on top. Season with salt and pepper to taste. Roast until the fennel is lightly colored and tender, turning twice, about 45 minutes.

Cook the linguine according to package directions and drain. Spoon the linguine into a large serving dish, and toss with the roasted vegetables and warm broth. Pass the Parmesan at the table.

Kilocalories 520 Kc • Protein 14 gm • Fat 17 gm • Percent of calories from fat 30% • Cholesterol 0 mg • Dietary fiber 6 gm • Sodium 128 mg • Calcium 55 mg

ANTIOXIDANT POWER

100

Ravioli with Chard

Often a first course at Italian holiday dinners, ravioli can be enhanced by combining it with antioxidant-rich vegetables like chard.

1 bunch Swiss chard (½ to ¾ pound)
1 tablespoon olive oil
2 garlic cloves, minced
2 cups tomato sauce (page 14 or use store-bought sauce from a jar)

4 dozen small frozen cheese-filled ravioli
½ cup freshly grated Parmesan cheese

Wash the chard well and trim off the stalk ends. Cut the stalks into ½-inch pieces and chop the leaves coarsely. Heat the oil in a large skillet and sauté the chard for 1 minute, stirring. Add the garlic and stir 1 minute longer. Add the tomato sauce, cover, and simmer until the chard is tender, about 5 minutes.

Cook the ravioli according to package directions; drain. Spoon half the chard mixture into a large pasta serving dish. Layer the ravioli on top. Spoon the remaining chard over all and sprinkle with the cheese.

Kilocalories 412 Kc • Protein 20 gm • Fat 18 gm • Percent of calories from fat 39% • Cholesterol 68 mg • Dietary fiber 5 gm • Sodium 761 mg • Calcium 296 mg

GRAINS, RICE, AND PASTA

Sweet Potatoes and Green Beans with Penne

---◼---

MAKES 4 SIDE-DISH SERVINGS

This colorful dish can accompany any meat course and complete the meal, combining as it does "something yellow and something green" with popular pasta.

2 large sweet potatoes, peeled and diced
½ pound fresh green beans, cut diagonally into 1-inch pieces
2 tablespoons olive oil
2 garlic cloves, minced
¼ teaspoon salt
Freshly ground black pepper

2 tablespoons chopped fresh basil or ½ teaspoon dried
8 ounces penne
About ½ cup low-sodium chicken or vegetable broth
2 ounces finely diced Asiago cheese

Cook the sweet potatoes in boiling salted water until tender, about 5 minutes. Remove with a slotted spoon. Cook the green beans in the same water until tender, 5 to 7 minutes. Drain.

Heat the oil in a large skillet and sauté the garlic until it's sizzling and fragrant, about 1 minute. Add the potatoes, green beans, salt, and pepper to taste, and stir-fry for 3 minutes to blend the flavors. Stir in the basil.

Cook the penne according to package directions and drain. Toss the penne gently with the vegetables and enough broth to moisten. Add the cheese and toss again.

Kilocalories 533 Kc • Protein 17 gm • Fat 13 gm • Percent of calories from fat 21% • Cholesterol 11 mg • Dietary fiber 6 gm • Sodium 442 mg • Calcium 271 mg

Fresh Tomato and Olive Sauce with Spaghetti

One of the joys of late summer is a savory sauce made with locally grown tomatoes and fresh basil.

3 tablespoons extra-virgin olive oil

2 garlic cloves, minced

5 cups vine-ripened tomatoes, peeled, seeded, and chopped (about 3 pounds)

¼ cup pitted chopped green olives

¼ cup pitted chopped black olives

¼ teaspoon salt

Freshly ground black pepper

¼ cup finely chopped fresh basil

1 pound spaghetti

Freshly grated Parmesan cheese

Heat the olive oil in a large skillet and sauté the garlic until it's soft and fragrant, about 1 minute. Add the tomatoes, olives, salt, and pepper to taste. Simmer, uncovered, stirring often, until the mixture reaches a sauce consistency, about 25 minutes. Stir in the basil and remove from the heat.

Cook the spaghetti according to package directions and drain. In a large serving dish, toss the spaghetti with the sauce. Pass the grated cheese at the table.

Kilocalories 615 Kc • Protein 18 gm • Fat 16 gm • Percent of calories from fat 23% • Cholesterol 0 mg • Dietary fiber 7 gm • Sodium 423 mg • Calcium 44 mg

GRAINS, RICE, AND PASTA

Fresh Tomato Sauce with Anchovies and Bell Peppers on Linguine

To keep the flavor and lose some of the salt in anchovies, rinse them in wine vinegar before adding them to the recipe.

3 tablespoons olive oil
3 garlic cloves, minced
1 green bell pepper, seeded
  and diced
1 red bell pepper, seeded
  and diced
1 (2-ounce) can anchovies,
  drained
1 dry hot red chili (optional)

5 cups vine-ripened tomatoes,
  peeled, seeded, and chopped
  (about 3 pounds)
¼ teaspoon freshly ground black
  pepper
2 tablespoons minced fresh flat-
  leaf parsley
1 tablespoon minced fresh basil
1 pound linguine

Heat the olive oil in a 12-inch skillet and sauté the garlic, bell peppers, anchovies, and chili, if using, over very low heat until the anchovies soften and break up, 5 to 7 minutes. Add the tomatoes and simmer over medium heat, uncovered, stirring often, until the mixture reaches a sauce consistency, 25 to 30 minutes. Remove and discard the chili. Stir in the black pepper, parsley, and basil.

Cook the linguine according to package directions and drain. Toss the linguine with the sauce.

Kilocalories 600 Kc • Protein 21 gm • Fat 14 gm • Percent of calories from fat 21% • Cholesterol 12 mg • Dietary fiber 6 gm • Sodium 420 mg • Calcium 76 mg

Fresh Tomato Sauce with Shrimp and Linguine

MAKES 4 SERVINGS

Tomatoes are especially rich in lycopene, a carotenoid member of the provitamin A family. Recent research has suggested that men who eat tomatoes, particularly the concentrated tomatoes cooked with oil in a sauce, are less at risk for prostate cancer.

¼ cup olive oil

1 dry hot red chili (optional)

2 shallots, minced

2 garlic cloves, minced

4 cups vine-ripened tomatoes, peeled, seeded, and chopped (about 2½ pounds)

4 strips lemon zest, no white pith

¼ teaspoon salt

Freshly ground black pepper

A few dashes of cayenne

¾ pound cooked shelled cleaned small shrimp (page 18 or use frozen, cooked shrimp thawed under running water)

¼ cup chopped fresh flat-leaf parsley

6 to 8 fresh basil leaves, slivered

1 pound thin linguine

Heat the olive oil in a large skillet and sauté the chili, shallots, and garlic until sizzling, about 1 minute. Add the tomatoes, lemon zest, salt, cayenne, and pepper to taste, and bring the sauce to a boil. Reduce the heat and simmer, uncovered, stirring often, until a sauce consistency is reached, 25 to 30 minutes. Add the shrimp, parsley, and basil. Keep the sauce warm for a few minutes to combine the flavors. Remove and discard the chili.

Cook the linguine according to package directions and drain. Spoon the linguine into a large serving dish and toss with some of the sauce. Pour the rest of the sauce on top and serve at once.

Kilocalories 665 Kc • Protein 34 gm • Fat 17 gm • Percent of calories from fat 22% • Cholesterol 166 mg • Dietary fiber 5 gm • Sodium 362 mg • Calcium 74 mg

GRAINS, RICE, AND PASTA

Fresh and Sun-dried Tomatoes, Chickpeas, and Penne

MAKES 4 SERVINGS

Vine-ripened tomatoes make a supereasy uncooked sauce for pasta.

¼ cup extra-virgin olive oil
1 large garlic clove, crushed
   through a press
4 cups vine-ripened tomatoes,
   unpeeled but seeded and diced
   (about 2½ pounds)
⅔ cup slivered oil-packed sun-
   dried tomatoes, drained
1 (14- to 16-ounce) can low-
   sodium chickpeas, drained and
   rinsed

2 tablespoons minced fresh flat-
   leaf parsley
1 tablespoon minced fresh basil
¼ teaspoon salt
Freshly ground black pepper
Hot red pepper flakes
1 pound penne or ziti
Freshly grated Parmesan cheese

In a medium bowl, mix the oil with the garlic. Stir in the fresh and dried tomatoes, chickpeas, parsley, basil, salt, and black and red peppers to taste. Allow the sauce to marinate at room temperature for a half hour or so.

Cook the penne according to package directions and drain. Spoon the penne into a large serving dish and toss with the sauce. Pass the Parmesan cheese at the table.

Kilocalories 780 Kc • Protein 26 gm • Fat 21 gm • Percent of calories from fat 24% • Cholesterol 0 mg • Dietary fiber 13 gm • Sodium 227 mg • Calcium 92 mg

Roasted Tomatoes and Onions with Asiago Cheese and Fusilli

MAKES 4 SERVINGS

We tend to think of the onion as a flavoring agent rather than as a vegetable all on its own, but in this pasta dish roasted onions take a starring role.

2 medium yellow onions
2 tablespoons olive oil
2 pounds plum tomatoes
¼ teaspoon salt
Freshly ground black pepper
1 teaspoon chopped fresh
   rosemary or ¼ teaspoon dried

12 ounces fusilli
½ cup warmed vegetable stock
   (page 11) or canned low-
   sodium broth
2 ounces Asiago cheese, very
   thinly slivered

Preheat the oven to 400 degrees F.

Peel and slice the onions into wedges about ½ inch at the thickest part. Put the onions in a large gratin pan, pour 1 tablespoon of oil over them, and stir to coat all sides. Bake until slightly softened, about 20 minutes.

Meanwhile, halve and seed the tomatoes. Add the tomatoes to the pan with the remaining tablespoon of oil and stir again. Season with the salt and pepper to taste, and sprinkle with the rosemary. Bake until the tomatoes and onions are both very tender, about 20 minutes.

Cook the fusilli according to package directions and drain. Toss the pasta with the vegetables and stock. If there's room, do this right in the gratin dish. Stir in the cheese and serve.

Kilocalories 522 Kc • Protein 20 gm • Fat 13 gm • Percent of calories from fat 23% • Cholesterol 11 mg • Dietary fiber 6 gm • Sodium 443 mg • Calcium 240 mg

Zucchini, Chilies, and Sun-dried Tomatoes with Shells

Chilies are sometimes overlooked as a great source of vitamin C.

2 tablespoons olive oil
1 medium zucchini, cut into
 1-inch chunks (½ to ¾ pound)
2 large Anaheim chilies, seeded
 and cut into 1-inch chunks
½ cup slivered oil-packed sun-
 dried tomatoes, drained
1 garlic clove, minced

1 tablespoon minced fresh
 cilantro or 1 teaspoon dried
½ teaspoon dried oregano
Freshly ground black pepper
8 ounces medium shell pasta
½ cup shredded Monterey Jack
 cheese

Heat the oil in a large skillet. Sauté the zucchini and chilies over medium-high heat until the zucchini begins to brown and is tender, about 5 minutes. Add the tomatoes and garlic. Lower the heat and continue to sauté for 3 minutes, stirring often. Add the cilantro, oregano, and pepper to taste.

Meanwhile, cook the shells according to package directions. Drain the shells, keeping them slightly moist, and spoon them into a large serving dish. Toss with the zucchini sauce. Sprinkle with the cheese and serve.

Kilocalories 683 Kc • Protein 28 gm • Fat 22 gm • Percent of calories from fat 28% • Cholesterol 10 mg • Dietary fiber 6 gm • Sodium 188 mg • Calcium 317 mg

Roasted Vegetables with Linguine

MAKES 4 SIDE-DISH SERVINGS, 2 MAIN-DISH SERVINGS

To choose a perfect eggplant, you have to "press the flesh." The eggplant should yield to your touch yet spring back resiliently when you release it.

2 small young eggplants, unpeeled (about 1 pound)
2 small zucchini (½ to ¾ pound)
4 plum tomatoes
1 green bell pepper
1 red bell pepper
2 tablespoons olive oil
2 garlic cloves, finely chopped
1 tablespoon minced fresh flat-leaf parsley
¼ teaspoon salt
Freshly ground black pepper
8 ounces linguine
½ pound diced part-skim mozzarella cheese
Hot red pepper flakes (optional)

Preheat the oven to 375 degrees F.

Trim off the ends of the eggplants and quarter them lengthwise. Cut the quarters into 1-inch pieces. Halve the zucchini lengthwise and cut the halves into 1-inch pieces. Cut the ends off the plum tomatoes and halve them lengthwise. Seed the bell peppers and cut them into 1-inch strips. In a large roasting pan, toss the vegetables with the oil and garlic. Arrange them in one layer and bake until they are quite tender, about 40 minutes. Turn the vegetables once or twice while they are roasting. Season the vegetables with parsley, salt, and pepper to taste.

Cook the linguine according to package directions and drain. In a large serving dish, toss the linguine with the vegetables and cheese. If desired, pass hot red pepper flakes at the table.

Kilocalories 452 Kc • Protein 30 gm • Fat 12 gm • Percent of calories from fat 23% • Cholesterol 16 mg • Dietary fiber 6 gm • Sodium 301 mg • Calcium 452 mg

GRAINS, RICE, AND PASTA

Rigatoni *Verdi*

3 tablespoons olive oil

1 fennel bulb, cored and sliced into 6 to 8 wedges

2 garlic cloves, minced

1 (9-ounce) package frozen artichoke hearts, thawed to separate

1 cup vegetable or chicken stock (pages 11, 10) or canned low-sodium broth

¼ teaspoon salt

¼ teaspoon freshly ground black pepper

⅛ teaspoon hot red pepper flakes

10 ounces fresh spinach, well washed, tough stems removed, coarsely chopped

12 ounces rigatoni

½ cup slivered Asiago cheese or ¼ cup slivered Parmesan cheese

Heat the oil in a Dutch oven and sauté the fennel until it's lightly colored, 5 to 7 minutes. Stir in the garlic and sauté 1 minute more. Add the artichoke hearts, stock, salt, and the black and red peppers. Cover and cook until the vegetables are tender, about 15 minutes. Add the spinach, cover, and cook until it wilts, 3 to 5 minutes.

Cook the rigatoni according to package directions and drain. Spoon the rigatoni into a large serving dish and toss with some of the vegetable pan juices. Ladle the rest of the vegetable mixture on top and sprinkle with the Asiago cheese.

Kilocalories 494 Kc • Protein 18 gm • Fat 14 gm • Percent of calories from fat 24% • Cholesterol 4 mg • Dietary fiber 8 gm • Sodium 383 mg • Calcium 197 mg

Chicken Primavera with Shells

MAKES 4 SERVINGS

1 broccoli crown (about
⅓ pound)
1 medium zucchini (about
½ pound)
1 red bell pepper
1 whole skinless boneless
chicken breast (about
¾ pound)
¼ cup unbleached all-
purpose flour
3 tablespoons olive oil

1 small yellow onion, chopped
1 garlic clove, minced
1 cup chicken stock (page 10) or
canned low-sodium broth
Salt and freshly ground black
pepper
2 tablespoons chopped fresh
flat-leaf parsley
1 tablespoon chopped fresh
basil or ½ teaspoon dried
12 ounces large shell pasta

Cut the broccoli into small florets and ½-inch pieces of stalk. Cut the zucchini into 1-inch chunks. Seed and cut the bell pepper into 1-inch chunks.

Wash the chicken in salted water, rinse, and pat it dry in paper towels.
Cut the chicken into 1-inch chunks. Put the flour in a plastic bag with the
chicken and shake to coat. Shake off excess flour.

Heat the oil in a 12-inch nonstick skillet and brown the chicken pieces
on all sides. Add the broccoli, zucchini, bell pepper, and onion, and stir-
fry until slightly softened, about 3 minutes. Add the garlic and stir-fry
1 minute longer. Add the stock, scraping the bottom of the pan as the
liquid boils up. Simmer, uncovered, stirring occasionally, until the vegetables are tender, the chicken is cooked through, and the sauce is slightly
thickened, about 8 minutes. Season with salt and pepper to taste (the
stock will add some salt). Stir in the parsley and basil. Keep the sauce
warm.

Cook the pasta according to package directions. Drain and transfer to a
large serving dish. Toss with the chicken and vegetables.

Kilocalories 570 Kc • Protein 34 gm • Fat 13 gm • Percent of calories from fat
21% • Cholesterol 50 mg • Dietary fiber 5 gm • Sodium 86 mg • Calcium 65 mg

GRAINS, RICE, AND PASTA

Chicken and Asparagus with Asian Noodles

Cashews are rich in vitamin E and folate, a B vitamin that works with antioxidants to help prevent cancer.

1 pound skinless boneless
  chicken breast
1 pound fresh asparagus
1 large red bell pepper
1 bunch scallions
1 tablespoon cornstarch
¾ cup chicken stock (page 10)
  or canned low-sodium broth
1 tablespoon naturally brewed
  reduced-sodium soy sauce

1 teaspoon sesame oil
½ teaspoon sugar
2 tablespoons canola or
  peanut oil
½ cup unsalted cashews
2 slices fresh ginger, minced
10 to 12 ounces fresh Asian
  noodles (linguine can be
  substituted)

Put the chicken in a freezer for a few minutes until it's firm. Thinly slice the partially frozen chicken. Trim off the woody ends of the asparagus and cut it diagonally into 2-inch pieces. Seed and cut the bell pepper into triangles. Cut the scallions into 1-inch pieces.

In a small pitcher or cup, blend the cornstarch with the stock, soy sauce, sesame oil, and sugar.

In a large wok or skillet, heat the oil and stir-fry the chicken, asparagus, bell pepper, scallions, cashews, and ginger until the chicken is cooked through and the asparagus is tender-crisp, 3 to 5 minutes. Add the stock mixture and stir constantly until it thickens and coats the chicken and vegetables.

Meanwhile, have a large pot of boiling salted water ready to cook the noodles according to package directions—fresh Asian noodles take only 1 to 2 minutes. (If you substitute dried linguine, start cooking it when you begin the stir-fry.) Drain and spoon the noodles into a large serving dish. Top with the chicken mixture.

Kilocalories 406 Kc • Protein 33 gm • Fat 18 gm • Percent of calories from fat 39% • Cholesterol 66 mg • Dietary fiber 4 gm • Sodium 241 mg • Calcium 68 mg

Shrimp, Peas, and Artichoke Hearts with Spinach Fettuccine

■

Recent research has found that shrimp does not raise cholesterol in the human body, as was previously thought to be the case.

2 tablespoons olive oil
1 to 2 garlic cloves, minced
¾ to 1 pound cooked shelled
  deveined shrimp (page 18 or
  use frozen cooked shrimp
  thawed)
2 cups fresh shelled or
  frozen peas
1 (9-ounce) package frozen
  artichoke hearts, thawed to
  separate

½ cup chicken stock (page 10)
  or canned low-sodium broth
2 tablespoons chopped fresh
  flat-leaf parsley
¼ teaspoon salt
Freshly ground black pepper
8 ounces spinach fettuccine
2 tablespoons fresh lemon juice

Heat the oil in a large skillet and sauté the garlic until it's sizzling and fragrant, 1 to 2 minutes. Add the shrimp and continue to sauté for 2 to 3 minutes. Remove the shrimp with a slotted spoon.

Add the peas, artichoke hearts, and stock to the pan. Cover and cook until the vegetables are tender, about 5 minutes. Return the shrimp to the pan. Season the dish with parsley, salt, and pepper to taste.

Meanwhile cook the fettuccine according to package directions and drain. Sprinkle the lemon juice over the shrimp mixture. Spoon the fettuccine into a large serving dish and toss with the shrimp and vegetables.

Kilocalories 346 Kc • Protein 21 gm • Fat 8 gm • Percent of calories from fat 21% • Cholesterol 61 mg • Dietary fiber 14 gm • Sodium 442 mg • Calcium 65 mg

GRAINS, RICE, AND PASTA

Spicy Pasta Salad with Vegetables

This is just the dish to take along on a picnic!

For the dressing

⅓ cup mayonnaise

½ cup nonfat plain yogurt

1 tablespoon fresh lemon juice

1 shallot, minced

1 garlic clove, crushed through
 a press

1 jalapeño chili, seeded and
 minced (wear rubber gloves)

1 teaspoon chili powder

½ teaspoon hot pepper sauce,
 such as Tabasco

½ teaspoon ground cumin

1 tablespoon chopped fresh
 cilantro

For the salad

1 broccoli crown, chopped
 (about ½ pound)

2 cups fresh or frozen corn
 kernels

½ pound green beans, cut into
 1-inch lengths

¼ teaspoon salt

1 small zucchini or cucumber,
 thinly sliced (¼ pound)

2 large ripe tomatoes, diced

8 ounces penne

Blend together the mayonnaise and yogurt. Stir in all the remaining dressing ingredients. Chill the dressing while making the salad.

Combine the broccoli, corn, green beans, 1 cup water, and salt in a saucepan, bring to a boil, and cook, covered, until the vegetables are tender-crisp, 3 to 5 minutes. Drain and rinse in cool water until the vegetables are no longer warm.

In a salad bowl, combine the cooked vegetables, zucchini, and tomatoes.

Meanwhile, cook the penne according to package directions. Drain and rinse in cool water. Stir into the vegetables. Blend in the dressing. Chill until ready to serve.

Kilocalories 314 Kc • Protein 10 gm • Fat 10 gm • Percent of calories from fat 27% • Cholesterol 8 mg • Dietary fiber 5 gm • Sodium 196 mg • Calcium 91 mg

Main Dishes

———————◼———————

The heart of the meal, the main dish, should have star quality. Whether it's a meat, fish, or vegetarian entrée, it needs to be both attractive and substantial. Complementary side dishes, salad, and bread may round out the meal, but main dishes must get the center stage. A main dish ought to be more than the chunk of meat that was so often served up in years past. Adding vegetables, legumes, grains, and vitamin E–rich oils enriches main dishes with the antioxidants that keep us healthy and vigorous, helping to reduce damage to the body from free radicals.

The main dishes in this chapter include poultry, meat, seafood, and egg entrées to which antioxidant foods have been added, and they also include a number of strictly vegetarian dishes that are inherently rich in antioxidant power. Even if you're not a vegetarian, it makes good health sense to enjoy a few meatless meals every week as a change of pace and a respite for your arteries.

Many of these main dishes—such as Oven-braised Chicken with Root Vegetables or Seafood Casserole with Broccoli or Vegetable Goulash—need little else to accompany them. They are entitled to that useful appellation "one-pot meal." Others require one or two supporting players—a great soup starter or a big salad on the side, plus the company of good fresh bread, preferably whole grain. Either way, they offer you a panoply of vitamins and minerals prepared in a taste-tempting way. Cook them up and serve them forth with the satisfying feeling that "this food *is* love."

Chicken with Carrots, Sweet Potatoes, and Peas

2 tablespoons olive oil

¼ cup chopped shallots

2 celery stalks, sliced

2 large carrots, diced

2 chicken breast quarters, skinned as much as possible (about 2 pounds)

1 very large or 2 medium sweet potatoes, peeled and halved lengthwise

2 cups chicken stock (page 10) or canned low-sodium broth

3 to 4 fresh sage and thyme sprigs

1 cup shelled fresh peas or frozen peas, thawed to separate

In a Dutch oven or other heavy pan, heat the oil and sauté the shallots, celery, and carrots until lightly colored, about 5 minutes. Add the chicken pieces, sweet potato, stock, and sage and thyme, and bring to a boil. Reduce the heat and simmer, covered, until the chicken is cooked through, about 25 minutes. Add the peas during the last 3 minutes.

With a slotted spoon, remove the chicken and vegetables. With a knife and fork, remove the chicken from the bone and cut it into rough chunks. Dice the sweet potato. Measure the broth, reserving 1 cup for this dish and saving the rest for soup another day. If necessary, reheat the chicken and vegetables with the reserved cup of broth. Transfer to a serving dish.

Kilocalories 415 Kc • Protein 57 gm • Fat 10 gm • Percent of calories from fat 23% • Cholesterol 132 mg • Dietary fiber 4 gm • Sodium 277 mg • Calcium 55 mg

ANTIOXIDANT POWER

116

Chicken with Two Peppers and Cannellini

MAKES 6 SERVINGS

Beans are a wonderful "meat stretcher."

2 tablespoons olive oil
1½ pounds skinless, boneless
 chicken breasts, cut into
 6 serving-size pieces
1 red bell pepper, seeded and
 cut into chunks
1 green bell pepper, seeded and
 cut into chunks
1 large sweet onion, chopped
1 cup chicken stock (page 10) or
 canned low-sodium broth
8 to 10 fresh sage leaves,
 chopped (about 1 tablespoon)

8 fresh basil leaves, chopped
 (about 1 tablespoon)
Freshly ground black pepper
2 cups homemade cannellini or
 white kidney beans (page 16)
 or canned low-sodium
 cannellini, drained and rinsed
1 tablespoon superfine flour,
 such as Wondra, stirred into
 ¼ cup cold water
Salt (optional)

In a Dutch oven or other heavy pan, heat the oil and brown the chicken pieces in batches. Remove the chicken and add the peppers and onion; sauté until slightly softened, 3 to 5 minutes. Return the chicken to the pan. Add the stock, sage, basil, and pepper to taste. Cover and simmer on low heat for 20 to 25 minutes, or until the chicken is just cooked through.

Add the beans and cook 5 minutes. Add the flour mixture and stir until the sauce bubbles and thickens, 2 to 3 minutes. Simmer 3 minutes. Taste the sauce to determine if it needs a little salt.

Kilocalories 276 Kc • Protein 33 gm • Fat 6 gm • Percent of calories from fat 21% • Cholesterol 66 mg • Dietary fiber 7 gm • Sodium 88 mg • Calcium 59 mg

MAIN DISHES

Chicken, Kale, and Corn Casserole

This is a wonderful make-ahead dish to stash in the refrigerator hours ahead of cooking time.

1 tablespoon olive oil
¼ cup chopped shallots or
  scallions
1 whole chicken breast, with or
  without bone, skinned (about
  1 pound boneless)
2 cups chicken stock (page 10)
  or canned low-sodium broth
1 teaspoon chopped fresh
  marjoram or
  ¼ teaspoon dried
1 fresh sage sprig
1 fresh thyme sprig

⅛ teaspoon freshly ground black
  pepper
2 cups chopped fresh or
  frozen kale
2 cups fresh or frozen corn
  kernels
1 tablespoon cornstarch
¼ cup cold water
Salt (optional)
1 cup crushed unsalted
  crackers
A few dashes of paprika

Heat the oil in a large saucepan and sauté the shallots until they begin to soften, 3 minutes. Add the chicken breast and brown it slightly. Add the broth, herbs, and pepper, and simmer until the chicken is cooked through, 15 to 20 minutes. Remove the chicken, bone it, and cut it into large chunks.

Cook the kale by simmering in the remaining broth until it's almost tender, 8 to 10 minutes; taste is the best test. Add the corn and cook an additional 3 minutes. Remove the vegetables with a slotted spoon and put them into a 2-quart gratin dish or casserole. Arrange the chicken on top. The recipe can be prepared ahead to this point and refrigerated.

Preheat the oven to 350 degrees F.

Measure the remaining broth; you should have 1 cup. If not, add enough water to make 1 cup; the broth will be concentrated and flavorful. Stir the cornstarch into the ¼ cup cold water and whisk it into the broth over high heat, stirring constantly, until the mixture bubbles and thickens, 2 to 3 minutes. Taste the sauce to see if you need salt. Pour the sauce over the chicken. Sprinkle with the crushed crackers and paprika. Bake until the crumbs are golden and the casserole is heated through, about 20 minutes (30 minutes if refrigerated).

Kilocalories 340 Kc • Protein 32 gm • Fat 7 gm • Percent of calories from fat 20% • Cholesterol 67 mg • Dietary fiber 3 gm • Sodium 246 mg • Calcium 79 mg

Acorn Squash Stuffed with Curried Chicken

MAKES 4 SERVINGS

This is a great dish for using up leftover cooked chicken or turkey.

2 large acorn squash
Ground nutmeg
1 tablespoon unsalted butter
1 tablespoon olive oil
2 teaspoons curry powder

1½ cups cooked cubed chicken (page 10)
1 Granny Smith apple, peeled, cored, and coarsely grated

Preheat the oven to 375 degrees F.

Cut the squash in half. Scoop out the seeds and strings. Sprinkle the flesh with a few dashes of nutmeg. Place the halves, cut sides up, in a roasting pan. Add ½ inch water. Bake the squash until they are tender, about 45 minutes.

Heat the butter and oil together in a medium skillet. Add the curry powder and cook for a minute or two, stirring. Blend in the chicken and apple.

Stuff the squash with the chicken mixture, mounding it up. Reduce the oven heat to 325 degrees F. Bake the squash until the chicken is heated through, about 20 minutes.

Kilocalories 244 Kc • Protein 18 gm • Fat 10 gm • Percent of calories from fat 36% • Cholesterol 53 mg • Dietary fiber 6 gm • Sodium 74 mg • Calcium 42 mg

Chicken Breasts with Braised Cabbage

MAKES 4 SERVINGS

Here's a supereasy skillet supper. Lightly cooked cabbage is rich in vitamin C.

2 tablespoons olive oil
4 chicken breast pieces,
  skinned, bone in (about
  1¼ pounds)
Salt and freshly ground black
  pepper
2 teaspoons chopped fresh
  thyme or ½ teaspoon dried

1 teaspoon chopped fresh
  rosemary or ¼ teaspoon dried
¼ cup chopped shallots
6 cups finely shredded green
  cabbage

Heat the oil in a 12-inch skillet and brown the chicken on one side. Turn and sprinkle with salt and pepper to taste and the herbs. Brown the second side, adding the shallots during the last 5 minutes. Put the pan cover on slightly ajar, and braise until the chicken is cooked through, 15 to 20 minutes for bone-in pieces.

Add the cabbage, which will seem like a lot, but heap it over the chicken—it will soon wilt. Cover the pan completely and cook 3 minutes. The cabbage should be wilted but tender-crisp. Remove the chicken, and stir the cabbage into the oil and juices at the bottom of the pan to catch all the good flavors. Cook 1 to 2 minutes more to the desired tenderness. Serve the cabbage with the chicken.

Kilocalories 242 Kc • Protein 34 gm • Fat 9 gm • Percent of calories from fat 33% • Cholesterol 82 mg • Dietary fiber 2 gm • Sodium 110 mg • Calcium 70 mg

ANTIOXIDANT POWER

120

Chicken, Sweet Potato, and Apricot Stew

MAKES 4 SERVINGS

Orange fruits as well as vegetables are rich in beta-carotene.

1½ pounds skinless chicken
  thighs, bone in
¼ cup unbleached all-
  purpose flour
2 tablespoons olive oil
1 medium yellow onion,
  chopped
1 garlic clove, minced
1 (1-pound) can Italian-style
  plum tomatoes with juice
½ cup or more chicken stock
  (page 10) or canned low-
  sodium broth

1 cinnamon stick
1 bay leaf
1 dry hot red chili
¼ teaspoon salt
Freshly ground black pepper
2 sweet potatoes, peeled and
  cut into 1-inch chunks (1 to
  1½ pounds)
8 dried apricots, halved

Put the chicken in a plastic bag with the flour. Hold the bag closed and shake to coat the chicken pieces. Shake off any excess flour.

In a Dutch oven or other heavy pan, heat the oil and brown the chicken in batches. Remove the chicken. Sauté the onion until soft and yellow, 3 to 5 minutes. Add the garlic during the last minute. Return the chicken to the pot. Add the tomatoes, stock, cinnamon stick, bay leaf, chili, and salt and pepper to taste. Cover and simmer for 10 minutes over low heat.

Add the sweet potatoes and apricots. Continue cooking until the potatoes are tender and the chicken is cooked through, 20 to 25 minutes more. Remove the cinnamon stick, bay leaf, and chili before serving.

Kilocalories 534 Kc • Protein 35 gm • Fat 20 gm • Percent of calories from fat 33% • Cholesterol 108 mg • Dietary fiber 8 gm • Sodium 279 mg • Calcium 101 mg

Chicken Cacciatore with Peas

■

Cacciatore simply means "hunter's style." Americans tend to "drown" chicken cacciatore in tomatoes, but this is not necessary to the authentic dish.

8 small skinless chicken thighs, with or without the bone
¼ cup olive oil
1 green bell pepper, seeded and cut into strips
1 red bell pepper, seeded and cut into strips
5 ounces mushrooms, cleaned and sliced
1 small yellow onion, chopped
2 garlic cloves, minced
½ cup dry vermouth or dry white wine
½ teaspoon dried oregano or basil
¼ teaspoon dried rosemary (optional—use if you like it)
¼ teaspoon salt
⅛ to ¼ teaspoon freshly ground black pepper
⅛ to ¼ teaspoon crushed hot red pepper flakes (optional)
1½ cups peeled chopped tomatoes or 1 (1-pound) can imported Italian tomatoes, drained (reserve the juice)
1½ cups shelled fresh or frozen peas
1 tablespoon minced fresh flat-leaf parsley

If the chicken is wet from washing, dry it on paper towels so that it won't splatter in the oil. Trim off any visible fat. Heat 2 tablespoons of oil in a Dutch oven and brown the chicken on both sides over medium-high heat in batches. Add a bit more oil if needed for the second batch. Remove the chicken.

Reduce the heat to medium. Add more oil as needed, and sauté the bell peppers, mushrooms, and onion, stirring often, until they are lightly colored, 3 to 5 minutes. Add the garlic and cook 1 minute longer. Add the vermouth, which will bubble up and begin to evaporate at once. Use this opportunity to scrape all the browned bits from the bottom of the pan.

Return the chicken to the pan. Add the oregano, rosemary if using, salt, and black and red peppers. Pour the tomatoes over all. Cook with the cover ajar over very low heat, stirring often, until the chicken is cooked through, about 20 minutes. If the sauce reduces too quickly, add a little of the reserved tomato juice. When the dish is finished, you should have 1 cup or less of sauce.

Add the peas, cover, and cook 5 minutes longer. Stir in the parsley.

Kilocalories 448 Kc • Protein 31 gm • Fat 25 gm • Percent of calories from fat 50% • Cholesterol 99 mg • Dietary fiber 5 gm • Sodium 361 mg • Calcium 37 mg

Oven-fried Chicken Breasts with Potatoes and Carrots

MAKES 4 SERVINGS

2 to 3 large russet potatoes
2 green bell peppers
1 large yellow onion
4 medium carrots
2 whole skinless, boneless
  chicken breasts

1 cup seasoned bread crumbs
  (see Note)
¼ cup toasted wheat germ
Milk (optional)
Salt and freshly ground black
  pepper

Preheat the oven to 375 degrees F.

Peel and cut the potatoes into quarters lengthwise. Seed and cut the peppers into 6 strips each. Peel and cut the onion into thick slices; separate the slices into rings. Cut each carrot into 3 pieces. Parboil the carrots in boiling salted water for 5 minutes; drain.

Cut each whole breast into 4 pieces. On a sheet of wax paper, mix the crumbs and wheat germ. If necessary, dampen the chicken with milk. Dip the chicken pieces in the crumbs to coat all sides.

Put the vegetables in a large oiled baking pan and bake in the middle of the oven for 20 minutes. Stir the vegetables, and season everything with salt and pepper to taste. Place the chicken pieces between them and bake for 10 minutes. Turn the chicken pieces and stir the vegetables again. Bake until the chicken is crusty, brown, and just cooked through and the vegetables are tender, about another 10 minutes.

NOTE: To coat chicken with seasoned crumbs, one very easy way is to reduce herb stuffing mix to fine crumbs in a food processor. The stuffing mix has a subtle herb seasoning that complements chicken.

To make homemade seasoned crumbs, mix 2 cups fine bread crumbs (made in a food processor) with ¼ teaspoon freshly ground black pepper, 1 teaspoon dried herbs of your choice, 1 tablespoon grated Parmesan cheese, and 2 tablespoons wheat germ. If you wish, 1 garlic clove crushed through a press can also be added. Spread the crumbs out on a baking sheet and toast them in a 300 degree F oven until dry and barely golden, about 20 minutes. This longer method has the advantage of being low in salt, and its fragrance when baking is divine!

Kilocalories 461 Kc • Protein 59 gm • Fat 4 gm • Percent of calories from fat 8% • Cholesterol 132 mg • Dietary fiber 7 gm • Sodium 226 mg • Calcium 74 mg

Oven-fried Chicken Breasts with Broccoli and Scallions

MAKES 4 SERVINGS

Not only high in antioxidant vitamins, broccoli is also a great source of calcium, fiber, and plant chemicals that guard against cancer.

2 red bell peppers
1 bunch scallions
1 pound broccoli crowns
2 whole skinless, boneless
  chicken breasts
1 cup seasoned bread crumbs
  (see Note, page 124)

¼ cup toasted wheat germ
Milk (optional)
Salt and freshly ground black
  pepper

Preheat the oven to 375 degrees F.

Seed and cut the peppers into 6 strips. Cut the scallions into 1-inch pieces. Cut the broccoli into thin (about ½-inch) stalks with florets attached. Parboil the broccoli in boiling salted water for 1 minute; drain.

Cut each whole breast into 4 pieces. On a sheet of wax paper, mix the crumbs and wheat germ. If necessary, dampen the chicken with milk. Dip the chicken pieces in the crumbs to coat all sides.

Put the chicken and vegetables in a large oiled baking pan and bake in the middle of the oven for 10 minutes. Stir the vegetables, turn the chicken, and season everything with salt and pepper to taste. Bake until the chicken is just cooked through and the vegetables are tender-crisp, 10 to 15 minutes more.

Kilocalories 341 Kc • Protein 59 gm • Fat 4 gm • Percent of calories from fat 11% • Cholesterol 132 mg • Dietary fiber 6 gm • Sodium 224 mg • Calcium 100 mg

Chicken Ragout with Artichoke Hearts

———————————■———————————

This chicken stew in the French style is reminiscent of Italian cacciatore. Rice is a nice accompaniment.

1 (28-ounce) can plum tomatoes in puree

1 tablespoon olive oil

1 tablespoon unsalted butter

½ cup chopped shallots

¼ teaspoon salt

¼ teaspoon freshly ground black pepper

1 teaspoon chopped fresh rosemary or ¼ teaspoon dried

1 teaspoon chopped fresh thyme or ¼ teaspoon dried

1 teaspoon chopped fresh tarragon or ¼ teaspoon dried

1¼ to 1½ pounds skinless, boneless chicken breasts, cut into 1-inch cubes

1 (9-ounce) package frozen artichoke hearts, thawed to separate

Put the tomatoes through a food mill to remove the seeds. Or you can scoop up each tomato, cut it in half, then seed and chop it by hand—a messy job, but it doesn't take long.

Heat the oil and butter in a large skillet, and sauté the shallots until they are sizzling, about 1 minute. Add the tomatoes and their puree, salt, pepper, and herbs. Simmer, uncovered, stirring often, for 10 minutes, until slightly reduced and "saucy."

Add the chicken and artichokes. Simmer, with the cover ajar, stirring often, until the chicken is cooked through but not dry and the artichokes are tender, 10 to 15 minutes.

Kilocalories 290 Kc • Protein 37 gm • Fat 7 gm • Percent of calories from fat 21% • Cholesterol 86 mg • Dietary fiber 7 gm • Sodium 324 mg • Calcium 116 mg

Chicken and Mixed Vegetable Salad

―――――――――― ■ ――――――――――

MAKES 4 SERVINGS—OR MORE IF PART OF A BUFFET

This is a wonderful summer supper dish to make early in the day. Chicken should be refrigerated as soon as possible after cooking.

1 whole skinless, boneless chicken breast, cut into 4 pieces (about ¾ pound)
¾ pound red potatoes, peeled and quartered
2 carrots, sliced
2 cups chicken stock (page 10) or canned low-sodium broth
1 tablespoon fresh lemon juice
½ pound fresh green beans, trimmed and cut into 1-inch pieces

2 celery stalks, diced
2 scallions, chopped
¼ cup mayonnaise
½ cup nonfat plain yogurt
¼ teaspoon dried dill
¼ teaspoon celery salt
¼ teaspoon white pepper
1 tablespoon chopped fresh flat-leaf parsley
8 small cherry tomatoes

Put the chicken, potatoes, and carrots into a saucepan with the stock and lemon juice. Bring to a boil, cover, and simmer until the vegetables are tender and the chicken is cooked through, 15 to 20 minutes. Scoop out the chicken and vegetables with a slotted spoon onto a large platter so they will cool more quickly. Use a knife and fork to dice the chicken and potatoes. Refrigerate promptly.

Cook the green beans in boiling salted water until they are tender-crisp, 5 to 7 minutes. Drain and rinse in cold water.

Combine the chicken, potatoes, carrots, green beans, celery, and scallions in a bowl. Whisk together the mayonnaise, yogurt, dill, celery salt, and pepper. Stir the dressing and fresh parsley into the salad. Garnish with the tomatoes. Chill until ready to serve.

Kilocalories 370 Kc • Protein 27 gm • Fat 13 gm • Percent of calories from fat 32% • Cholesterol 60 mg • Dietary fiber 6 gm • Sodium 207 mg • Calcium 121 mg

MAIN DISHES

Oven-braised Chicken with Root Vegetables

---■---

MAKES 6 SERVINGS

The chicken for this dish is a young broiler-fryer left whole; it will cook quickly and be less fatty than a large roaster. This is one of the easiest "company dinners" ever, a real bonus.

1 (3½- to 4-pound) whole chicken
1 (4-inch) fresh rosemary sprig
1 garlic clove, halved
1 tablespoon olive oil
1 tablespoon unsalted butter
3 Yukon Gold or red potatoes, peeled and halved

6 whole small shallots, peeled
6 whole small turnips, peeled
6 whole small carrots
Salt and freshly ground black pepper

Preheat the oven to 375 degrees F.

Wash the chicken in cold salted water; drain. Remove any internal lump of fat. Put the rosemary and garlic into the cavity, fold back the wings, and truss the chicken. In a large enameled cast-iron casserole, heat the oil with the butter. When the butter has melted, brown the chicken on one side, about 4 minutes, next on the other side, then the front breast. Turn the chicken upright and brown the back. Remove the chicken.

Put the vegetables in the pot and brown them lightly, turning often, 3 to 5 minutes. Remove the vegetables with a slotted spoon and return the chicken to the pot. Surround and top the chicken with the vegetables. (All this shifting is necessary to give everything a nice color and flavor and to end with the chicken on the bottom.) Season everything with salt and pepper to taste. Cover and bake about 1 hour. The chicken is cooked if the juices run clear when a thigh is pierced. The vegetables should be quite tender, too.

Transfer the chicken to a large platter and arrange the vegetables on another.

Kilocalories 664 Kc • Protein 66 gm • Fat 37 gm • Percent of calories from fat 51% • Cholesterol 262 mg • Dietary fiber 3 gm • Sodium 250 mg • Calcium 71 mg

Spiced Apricot Chicken with Lentils

Couscous would be a pleasing companion dish for this easy one-pot dinner with a Middle Eastern flavor.

2 tablespoons peanut or any vegetable oil
8 small skinless chicken thighs
1 large yellow onion, chopped
1 garlic clove, minced
1¾ cups chicken stock (page 10) or canned low-sodium broth
½ cup brown lentils, rinsed
1 large carrot, sliced
4 to 6 slivers orange rind
½ cup snipped dried apricots
½ teaspoon ground ginger
½ teaspoon ground coriander
¼ teaspoon ground cinnamon
Salt (optional)

Preheat the oven to 350 degrees F.

In a flameproof casserole, heat the oil and brown the chicken on both sides in batches over medium-high heat. Remove the chicken, reduce the heat, and sauté the onion until soft and lightly colored, 3 to 5 minutes. Add the garlic during the last minute. Return the chicken to the casserole.

Add the stock, lentils, carrot, orange rind, apricots, ginger, coriander, cinnamon, and salt, if using. Bring to a boil, stir gently, and cover. Set the casserole, covered and still simmering, in the middle of the oven and bake until the chicken is cooked and the lentils are just tender, about 40 minutes. Taste to determine if the lentils need more salt.

Kilocalories 438 Kc • Protein 37 gm • Fat 18 gm • Percent of calories from fat 38% • Cholesterol 100 mg • Dietary fiber 10 gm • Sodium 113 mg • Calcium 50 mg

Turkey and White Bean Chili

This is a spicy way to use leftover cooked turkey after the holidays.

2 tablespoons olive oil
1 large yellow onion, chopped
2 Anaheim chilies, seeded
   and diced
¾ to 1 pound turkey, cooked
   and diced or uncooked, cut
   into bite-size pieces
1 cup chicken or turkey stock
   (page 10) or canned low-
   sodium broth
¼ cup low-sodium tomato paste
1 teaspoon chili powder

1 teaspoon ground cumin
1 teaspoon fresh oregano or
   ¼ teaspoon dried
Freshly ground black pepper
½ teaspoon or more hot pepper
   sauce, such as Tabasco
1½ cups homemade white navy
   beans (page 16) or canned low-
   sodium navy beans, drained
   and rinsed
2 cups hot cooked brown rice

Heat the oil in a medium pot, and sauté the onion and chilies until soft-ened, 5 minutes. Add the turkey, and if it's uncooked, brown it. Add the stock, tomato paste, chili powder, cumin, and oregano. Stir in black pep-per and hot pepper sauce to taste. Simmer the mixture for 8 to 10 minutes for leftover cooked turkey, or until cooked through, about 15 minutes for raw turkey.

Stir in the beans and simmer a few minutes longer. Serve the turkey chili with hot cooked rice.

Kilocalories 433 Kc • Protein 29 gm • Fat 14 gm • Percent of calories from fat 29% • Cholesterol 49 mg • Dietary fiber 10 gm • Sodium 72 mg • Calcium 82 mg

Turkey Loaf with Shell Beans

A "heart" of shell beans makes this meat loaf richer in nutrients without adding fat.

1 large shallot, peeled and quartered
1 thick slice white Italian bread
¼ cup toasted wheat germ
2 tablespoons grated Parmesan cheese
1 tablespoon finely chopped fresh flat-leaf parsley
¼ teaspoon chopped fresh rosemary or a pinch of the dried herb

¼ teaspoon salt
¼ teaspoon freshly ground black pepper
1¼ pounds lean ground turkey
1 egg
1½ cups cooked or canned low-sodium shell beans, drained and rinsed
1 cup tomato sauce (page 14 or use store-bought sauce from a jar)

Preheat the oven to 350 degrees F.

Processor method: With the motor running, toss the shallot down the feed tube to mince it. Add the bread, torn into chunks, and process until it's crumbed. Blend in the wheat germ, cheese, herbs, and seasonings. Add the ground meat and egg, and process just long enough to blend.

By hand: Finely chop the shallots. Soften the bread in a little warm water, squeeze out excess moisture, and break it into pieces. Put all the ingredients into a bowl and mix with your hands, taking care to blend in the bread.

Put half the meat mixture into a loaf pan, smoothing it into a layer that is slightly higher at the edges. Add the beans and smooth the remaining meat over them. Top with the tomato sauce. Bake the meat loaf for 45 minutes, or until a thermometer inserted in the center registers 175 to 180 degrees F. Let rest 10 minutes. Carefully pour off the accumulated juices and slice into 6 slices.

Kilocalories 280 Kc • Protein 25 gm • Fat 12 gm • Percent of calories from fat 39% • Cholesterol 111 mg • Dietary fiber 6 gm • Sodium 295 mg • Calcium 78 mg

Veal Marsala with Peppers and Polenta

■

A cool green salad and crusty bread are all you need to complete this easy but elegant dinner. Technique is important to cooking this dish successfully, so try it once before making it for company. The polenta can be prepared a few hours or the day ahead, and the rest will go quite quickly.

1¼ to 1½ pounds veal scallops or turkey cutlets
Unbleached all-purpose flour
1 batch polenta (page 12), spread on a platter and chilled
3 tablespoons olive oil, or more as needed
3 bell peppers, seeded and cut into strips (if possible, use 3 different colors)

2 tablespoons balsamic vinegar
¼ teaspoon salt
Freshly ground black pepper
¾ cup chicken stock (page 10) or canned low-sodium broth
2 tablespoons fresh lemon juice
¼ cup marsala wine or dry vermouth
1 tablespoon minced fresh flat-leaf parsley

Put the veal scallops between sheets of wax paper and pound them with a wooden mallet or rolling pin until they are very thin, about ⅛ inch thick. Lightly dust them with flour.

Cut the polenta into 8 squares, put them on an oiled baking sheet, and heat them in a warm (250 degree F) oven about 20 minutes or until hot.

Heat 2 tablespoons of oil in a 12-inch skillet and sauté the peppers until they are tender-crisp, about 5 minutes. Remove them with a slotted spoon. Toss them with the vinegar, salt, and pepper to taste. Keep the peppers warm in the oven.

Add 1 tablespoon oil to the pan (plus more as needed), heat until medium-hot, and sauté the veal or turkey scallops, with plenty of room between them, in batches, until they are golden on both sides, about 2 minutes per side. Remove the scallops.

Add the stock, lemon juice, and marsala to the pan, and cook over high heat, watching carefully, until the mixture is reduced to half of its original volume and is slightly thickened, 3 to 5 minutes. There won't be much sauce but it has great concentrated flavor. Return the veal scallops to the pan, turning them over in the sauce, and rewarm them.

Divide the veal among 4 warm plates, spoon the pan sauce over them, and sprinkle with parsley. Put the polenta on the side and spoon the peppers on top.

Kilocalories 546 Kc • Protein 49 gm • Fat 20 gm • Percent of calories from fat 34% • Cholesterol 152 mg • Dietary fiber 4 gm • Sodium 440 mg • Calcium 160 mg

Oven-cooked Veal Stew with Sweet Potatoes

■

MAKES 4 SERVINGS

This stew is a powerhouse of vegetables rich in carotenes: sweet potatoes, carrots, and red bell peppers.

1½ pounds veal stew meat or boneless chicken breast in 1- to ¾-inch cubes, well trimmed

⅓ cup unbleached all-purpose flour

2 tablespoons or more olive oil

1 large red bell pepper, seeded and cut into 1-inch triangles

1 medium yellow onion, chopped

2 garlic cloves, finely chopped

2 cups chicken stock (page 10) or canned low-sodium broth

2 large sweet potatoes, peeled and cut into 1-inch pieces

2 large carrots, sliced diagonally into 1-inch pieces

1 cup "kitchen-ready" or crushed canned tomatoes

1 tablespoon chopped fresh marjoram or 1 teaspoon dried

Freshly ground black pepper

Salt (optional)

Preheat the oven to 375 degrees F.

Put the veal in a plastic bag with the flour and shake it to coat the meat. Shake off any excess flour. Heat the oil until quite hot in a Dutch oven and brown the meat in batches on all sides. Remove the meat and lower the heat.

Adding more oil if needed, sauté the bell pepper and onion 2 to 3 minutes, until sizzling and fragrant, and add the garlic during the last minute. Add the broth and scrape up all the browned bits from the bottom of the pan. Add the potatoes, carrots, tomatoes, marjoram, and pepper to taste. When the stew is simmering, give it a good stir and put it into the oven. Cook, covered, until everything is quite tender, about 45 minutes, stirring once during the cooking time. The flour on the meat will thicken the gravy, so this is really a one-step stew. Taste the gravy to determine if it needs salt.

Kilocalories 388 Kc • Protein 32 gm • Fat 13 gm • Percent of calories from fat 32% • Cholesterol 112 mg • Dietary fiber 5 gm • Sodium 138 mg • Calcium 71 mg

Pork Chops Normandy with Cabbage and Sweet Potatoes

MAKES 4 SERVINGS

Here's a one-dish meal that's a cinch to prepare. I like the cross-cultural touch of Bell Pepper Corn Bread (page 273) as an accompaniment.

1 tablespoon olive oil
¼ cup chopped shallots
4 large boneless pork chops or
   large skinless chicken thighs,
   well trimmed
2 large sweet potatoes, peeled
   and cut into 1-inch slices
Salt and freshly ground black
   pepper

½ cup dry white wine
½ cup chicken stock (page 10)
   or canned low-sodium broth
2 red apples
2 cups shredded green cabbage
1 scant teaspoon sugar
Dashes of ground cinnamon

Preheat the oven to 350 degrees F.

In a large skillet, heat the oil, add the shallots to the pan, and brown the pork chops on both sides, about 2 minutes per side. Transfer the chops to a 2½-quart gratin dish. Surround them with the potatoes. Salt and pepper everything to taste.

Add the wine and stock to the skillet and scrape up any browned bits. Pour the wine mixture over the chops. Cover and bake the dish in the middle of the oven for 25 minutes.

While the pork is cooking, core and slice the apples; do not peel them. Remove the dish from the oven and sprinkle the cabbage on top of the chops. Layer the apple rings in overlapping slices on top. Sprinkle the apples with sugar and cinnamon. Cover and continue baking for 15 minutes, or until everything is cooked through.

Kilocalories 253 Kc • Protein 24 gm • Fat 6 gm • Percent of calories from fat 23% • Cholesterol 61 mg • Dietary fiber 3 gm • Sodium 60 mg • Calcium 53 mg

Oven-fried Sole with Creamy Spinach

Actually, there's not an ounce of cream in this smooth, rich sauce.

8 fillets of sole (about
  1½ pounds total)
½ cup unbleached all-
  purpose flour
¾ cup seasoned dry bread
  crumbs
1 large egg
½ teaspoon salt
2 to 3 dashes of cayenne to taste
1 pound fresh spinach, washed,
  stemmed, and coarsely
  chopped

¼ cup stock, broth, or water
3 tablespoons nonfat dry milk
  powder
3 tablespoons superfine flour,
  such as Wondra
⅛ teaspoon freshly ground black
  pepper
Dash of ground nutmeg
1 cup low-fat milk
2 tablespoons fresh lemon juice
2 teaspoons olive oil
4 lemon wedges for garnish

Rinse and pat dry the fillets. Put the all-purpose flour on a sheet of wax paper and the crumbs on another. In a shallow soup bowl, beat the egg with 3 tablespoons of water, ¼ teaspoon of salt, and cayenne. Using 2 forks, coat the fish with the flour, then the egg mixture, then the crumbs. Chill the coated fish.

Put the spinach into a large pot with the stock and simmer until it wilts, about 5 minutes. Whisk the dry milk, superfine flour, the remaining ¼ teaspoon salt, black pepper, and nutmeg into the liquid milk. Add the milk mixture to the spinach, and stir until the sauce bubbles and thickens, about 3 minutes. Stir in the lemon juice. Simmer 3 minutes. Keep the spinach warm or reheat when the fish is ready.

Preheat the oven to 450 degrees F.

Place the fish on an oiled baking sheet and drizzle the fillets with 1 teaspoon of oil. Bake on the top shelf of the oven for 5 minutes. Carefully turn the fish with a spatula, drizzle with the remaining 1 teaspoon oil, and bake until golden and cooked through, about 5 more minutes.

To serve, divide the creamed spinach among 4 dinner plates. Place the fillets on top and garnish with lemon wedges.

Kilocalories 389 Kc • Protein 51 gm • Fat 8 gm • Percent of calories from fat 19% • Cholesterol 173 mg • Dietary fiber 4 gm • Sodium 647 mg • Calcium 246 mg

Fillet of Sole Roll-ups with Carrot Filling

MAKES 4 SERVINGS

An asparagus or broccoli salad (page 302) goes along nicely with this festive and easy dish.

1 large carrot
1 scallion, coarsely chopped
½ cup seasoned bread crumbs
   or cracker crumbs
¼ cup toasted wheat germ

¼ teaspoon dried basil
8 small fillets of sole (about
   1¼ pounds)
About 1 tablespoon olive oil

Preheat the oven to 400 degrees F.

In a food processor, mince the carrot and scallion. Briefly mix in the crumbs, wheat germ, and basil. Rinse the fillets and pat dry with paper towels. Stuff each with a heaping spoonful of the carrot mixture and roll it up. Place the rolls, seam side down, in an oiled baking dish. (If necessary, secure the rolls with toothpicks.) A little stuffing should be left over; sprinkle it on top of the rolls and drizzle with olive oil.

Bake the rolls in the top third of the oven until they flake apart easily, 18 to 20 minutes. (If you've used toothpicks, remove them before serving.)

Kilocalories 203 Kc • Protein 29 gm • Fat 6 gm • Percent of calories from fat 26% • Cholesterol 75 mg • Dietary fiber 2 gm • Sodium 144 mg • Calcium 33 mg

Broiled Swordfish with Warm Tomato Salad

Simple steamed broccoli would be an attractive side dish.

2 tablespoons olive oil
¼ cup chopped shallots
1 garlic clove, minced
2 cups peeled seeded chopped
   tomatoes
¼ teaspoon salt
⅛ teaspoon freshly ground black
   pepper

2 tablespoons red wine vinegar
1 tablespoon chopped fresh
   basil or 1 teaspoon dried
Dashes of hot pepper sauce,
   such as Tabasco
4 swordfish portions, about
   6 ounces each

Heat the oil in a medium skillet and sauté the shallots until they are softened, 3 minutes. Add the garlic and cook 1 minute longer. Add the tomatoes, salt, and pepper, and sauté for 3 minutes, stirring often. The tomatoes should keep their shape. Remove from the heat and stir in the vinegar, basil, and hot pepper sauce to taste.

Preheat the broiler. Place the swordfish steaks on an oiled baking sheet and broil them 6 inches from the heat for about 5 minutes per side, until they are cooked through. Arrange the swordfish on 4 dinner plates. If necessary, rewarm the salad. Top the swordfish with the tomato mixture, dividing it among the portions.

Kilocalories 244 Kc • Protein 28 gm • Fat 13 gm • Percent of calories from fat 46% • Cholesterol 53 mg • Dietary fiber 1 gm • Sodium 276 mg • Calcium 14 mg

ANTIOXIDANT POWER

Baked Haddock with Italian Peppers

Fish is so easy to prepare and quickly cooked, it qualifies as a home-made "fast food."

1 tablespoon olive oil
4 Italian frying peppers, seeded
  and chopped
4 scallions, chopped
1 large haddock fillet (1¼ to
  1½ pounds)

1 cup tomato sauce (page 14 or
  use store-bought sauce from
  a jar)
½ cup herb stuffing mix

Set the oven at 400 degrees F. Spread the oil in the bottom of a baking dish that will fit the fish fillet. Scatter the peppers and scallions over the oil, and put the dish in the oven while it's preheating. Bake until the vegetables are sizzling, 5 to 7 minutes. Remove the pan from the oven.

Carefully (because the pan is hot) lay the fish, skin side down, over the peppers. If one end of the fillet is thinner than the other, fold it under. Spread the sauce over the fillet. Scatter the stuffing mix over the sauce and press it down lightly. Bake until the fish flakes apart at the center, 15 to 20 minutes. If the crumbs get brown too fast, cover the pan loosely with foil.

Kilocalories 265 Kc • Protein 30 gm • Fat 9 gm • Percent of calories from fat 31% • Cholesterol 81 mg • Dietary fiber 3 gm • Sodium 250 mg • Calcium 88 mg

MAIN DISHES

139

Poached Haddock with Indian Cauliflower

■

Poaching is a technique that requires very low heat to create an extremely gentle simmer. Once you cover the pan, the heat accumulates under the lid, so lift it occasionally to make certain the simmer isn't escalating to a boil.

2 tablespoons peanut or any
   vegetable oil
1 small yellow onion, chopped
½ teaspoon ground cumin
½ teaspoon ground coriander
½ teaspoon ground ginger
¼ teaspoon cayenne
2 teaspoons cornstarch
1 cup vegetable stock (page 11)
   or canned low-sodium broth

½ large cauliflower, separated
   into florets (cut large florets
   in half)
1 large sweet potato, peeled and
   cut into 1-inch chunks
1½ pounds haddock, rinsed and
   cut into 4 pieces

In a 12-inch skillet, heat the oil and sauté the onion until it's lightly colored, 3 to 5 minutes. Add the cumin, coriander, ginger, and cayenne, and stir-fry for 1 minute. Whisk the cornstarch into the stock. Add the stock to the skillet and stir to blend the spices evenly. Keep stirring until the sauce thickens slightly. Add the cauliflower and sweet potato. Simmer, covered, until the vegetables are almost tender, about 5 minutes. Put the haddock on top and baste it with the sauce. Bring the sauce to a simmer, cover, and poach over very low heat until the haddock flakes apart easily and the vegetables finish cooking, about 5 minutes.

Kilocalories 286 Kc • Protein 35 gm • Fat 8 gm • Percent of calories from fat 27% • Cholesterol 97 mg • Dietary fiber 4 gm • Sodium 153 mg • Calcium 91 mg

Baked Scrod with Bell Peppers

MAKES 4 SERVINGS

Sweet white scrod is a New England favorite that lends itself to simple dishes like this one.

1 tablespoon olive oil
2 bell peppers (preferably different colors), seeded and cut into strips
1 yellow onion, halved and thinly sliced
Salt and freshly ground black pepper

1 large scrod fillet (1¼ to 1½ pounds)
¼ cup nonfat plain yogurt
¼ cup seasoned dry bread crumbs
2 tablespoons grated Parmesan cheese

Preheat the oven to 400 degrees F.

Spread the oil in the bottom of a baking dish that will fit the fish fillet. Scatter the bell peppers and onion over the oil, tossing to coat the vegetables. Season them with salt and pepper to taste.

Lay the fish, skin side down, over the peppers. If one end of the fillet is thinner than the other, fold it under. Spread the yogurt over the fillet. Scatter the crumbs over the yogurt and press down lightly. Sprinkle with the cheese. Bake until the fish flakes apart at the center, 15 to 20 minutes. If the crumbs get brown too fast, cover the pan loosely with foil.

Kilocalories 194 Kc • Protein 28 gm • Fat 5 gm • Percent of calories from fat 25% • Cholesterol 63 mg • Dietary fiber 1 gm • Sodium 145 mg • Calcium 98 mg

MAIN DISHES

Mediterranean Kedgeree

MAKES **2** SERVINGS

This is a great way to use leftover fish from any of the three preceding recipes.

⅓ to ½ pound cooked fish (plus whatever went with it, such as bell peppers)

2 cups cooked white or brown rice

2 tablespoons freshly grated Parmesan cheese

1 tablespoon olive oil

½ teaspoon dried Italian herbs, or a mixture of dried basil, oregano, and rosemary

Preheat the oven to 325 degrees F.

With a fork, separate the fish into large flakes and gently mix it (and whatever vegetables were cooked with it) with the rice and 1 tablespoon of the cheese. Spoon the mixture into an oiled 9-inch-square pan. Drizzle with the olive oil. Sprinkle the remaining 1 tablespoon of cheese on top. Sprinkle with the herbs. Bake until the cheese is melted and the dish is heated through, 20 to 25 minutes.

Kilocalories 390 Kc • Protein 21 gm • Fat 9 gm • Percent of calories from fat 22% • Cholesterol 47 mg • Dietary fiber 1 gm • Sodium 144 mg • Calcium 105 mg

Tuna with Cannellini

The mild taste of cannellini beans goes well with assertive tuna and Dijon mustard.

1½ pounds tuna steak
2 teaspoons Dijon mustard
1 cup fresh bread crumbs from
  1 slice Italian bread
Freshly ground black pepper
Paprika
1 tablespoon olive oil
1 red bell pepper, seeded
  and diced

2 garlic cloves, minced
2 cups homemade cannellini or
  white kidney beans (page 16)
  or 1 (14- to 16-ounce) can low-
  sodium cannellini, drained and
  rinsed
1 tablespoon minced fresh
  cilantro or parsley

Preheat the oven to 400 degrees F.

Oil a baking pan and place the tuna in it. Spread the top with mustard and sprinkle with bread crumbs. Season with pepper to taste. Sprinkle with paprika. Bake the fish in the top third of the oven until it's cooked through, about 18 minutes. If the crumbs appear to be getting too brown, lay a sheet of foil loosely over the top. Remove and let stand for 5 minutes.

Meanwhile, heat the oil in a medium skillet and sauté the pepper until it is softened, 5 minutes. Add the garlic and cook 1 minute. Add the beans and simmer 5 minutes. Stir in the cilantro or parsley.

Divide the beans among 4 warm dinner plates. Slice the tuna and arrange on top.

Kilocalories 354 Kc • Protein 44 gm • Fat 12 gm • Percent of calories from fat 32% • Cholesterol 65 mg • Dietary fiber 4 gm • Sodium 129 mg • Calcium 50 mg

Grilled Tuna Kebabs with Vegetables

Metal skewers get burning hot, so it's best to remove kebabs from them before serving.

¼ cup olive oil
¼ cup lemon juice
1 garlic clove, minced
1 slice fresh ginger, minced
¼ teaspoon dried thyme
¼ teaspoon salt
10 ounces button mushrooms, cleaned and stemmed (reserve the stems for another use)

1 large red bell pepper, seeded and cut into 1-inch chunks
1 to 1¼ pounds tuna steak, 1 inch thick, cut into 1½-inch cubes
8 to 12 cherry tomatoes
4 cups hot cooked brown rice
4 lemon wedges

In a shallow bowl, stir together the oil, lemon juice, garlic, ginger, thyme, and salt. Stir the mushrooms, bell pepper, and tuna into this mixture. Let the fish and vegetables marinate at room temperature for 20 minutes.

Thread the tuna, mushrooms, bell pepper, and cherry tomatoes on four 10-inch metal skewers. Grill the kebabs on an oiled rack 6 inches from glowing coals, or lay them on a broiler pan and broil under a preheated broiler. Turn from time to time while cooking. Remove when the tuna is cooked through, about 10 minutes.

To serve, divide the rice among 4 warm dinner plates. Gently push the contents of each skewer onto a plate of rice. Garnish with lemon wedges.

Kilocalories 537 Kc • Protein 33 gm • Fat 21 gm • Percent of calories from fat 35% • Cholesterol 43 mg • Dietary fiber 5 gm • Sodium 198 mg • Calcium 39 mg

ANTIOXIDANT POWER

Baked Red Snapper with Pinto Beans and Spinach

MAKES 4 SERVINGS

This is a complete dinner you can have ready in a half hour. Crusty French bread or corn bread would be good companions.

1 cup herb stuffing
2 tablespoons olive oil
4 scallions, chopped
4 red snapper fillets (6 to 7 ounces each)
¼ to ⅓ cup nonfat plain yogurt
Paprika
2 plum tomatoes, chopped
1 (14-ounce) package frozen pinto beans, thawed

1 tablespoon chopped fresh marjoram or 1 teaspoon dried oregano
¼ teaspoon hot red pepper flakes
2 garlic cloves, minced
1 pound fresh spinach, washed, stemmed, and coarsely chopped
Salt and freshly ground black pepper

In a food processor, reduce the stuffing mix to coarse crumbs.

Put 1 tablespoon oil in a baking pan that will hold the fish fillets in a single layer. Scatter the scallions over the bottom of the pan. Preheat the oven to 400 degrees F. While it's heating, put the pan in the oven until the scallions are sizzling, about 5 minutes. Remove the pan.

Rinse and pat dry the fillets. Turn them over in the pan to coat both sides with the scallion oil (carefully, since the pan may still be hot) and arrange them skin sides down. Spread with the yogurt and top with the stuffing crumbs. Sprinkle with paprika. Bake in the top third of the oven until cooked through, 18 to 20 minutes.

Mix the tomatoes, beans, marjoram, and hot pepper flakes in a small casserole, and heat them in the oven while the fish is cooking.

Meanwhile, heat the remaining tablespoon of oil in a large pot. Add the garlic and spinach, and stir-fry until the spinach wilts a bit. Add ½ cup water, cover, and simmer until cooked, 5 minutes. Drain and season with salt and pepper to taste.

Divide the spinach among 4 warm dinner plates. Top with the fish fillets. Divide the beans on the side.

Kilocalories 492 Kc • Protein 50 gm • Fat 11 gm • Percent of calories from fat 19% • Cholesterol 63 mg • Dietary fiber 13 gm • Sodium 496 mg • Calcium 275 mg

Poached Salmon with New Potatoes and Peas

■

MAKES 4 SERVINGS

This is a favorite Fourth of July dish with the traditional, but lighter, egg sauce.

2 large eggs	About 1 cup low-fat milk
1 tablespoon olive oil	½ cup nonfat dry milk powder
¼ cup chopped shallots	¼ cup superfine flour, such as
4 salmon steaks (about	Wondra
6 ounces each)	½ teaspoon celery salt
1 (8-ounce) bottle clam juice	¼ teaspoon white pepper
8 new potatoes, unpeeled, halved	2 teaspoons chopped fresh dill
8 baby carrots	or ½ teaspoon dried
1 cup vegetable or chicken stock	1 tablespoon chopped fresh
(page 11, 10) or canned low-	chives
sodium broth	Fresh dill sprigs for garnish
1 tablespoon fresh lemon juice	(optional)
2 cups shelled fresh or	
frozen peas	

Hard-boil the eggs. Cool, peel, and chop them.

In a 12-inch skillet, heat the oil and sauté the shallots until softened, about 3 minutes. Place the steaks on top and add the clam juice. Cover and cook at the lowest simmer until the salmon just flakes apart, about 8 minutes. Use a spatula to gently remove the salmon to a platter. Keep warm.

Separately simmer the potatoes and carrots in the stock and lemon juice, covered, until they are nearly tender, about 10 minutes. Add the peas and continue simmering until all the vegetables are tender, about 5 more minutes. Drain, reserving the broth. Keep the vegetables warm.

Combine the pan juices from the salmon and the stock in which the vegetables were cooked. Add ¼ cup milk and pour this mixture into a saucepan. Heat but do not boil the mixture yet. In a small pitcher, whisk the dry milk, flour, celery salt, and white pepper into the remaining ¾ cup cold milk. Pour this all at once into the saucepan, and stir constantly over medium heat until bubbling and thickened, about 5 minutes. Stir the dill into the sauce and continue to simmer for 3 minutes, stirring often. Remove from the heat and stir in the eggs and chives.

Serve the salmon surrounded by the vegetables and topped with some of the egg sauce. If desired, garnish with dill sprigs. Pass extra egg sauce in a pitcher.

Kilocalories 544 Kc • Protein 48 gm • Fat 19 gm • Percent of calories from fat 31% • Cholesterol 204 mg • Dietary fiber 7 gm • Sodium 194 mg • Calcium 184 mg

Baked Salmon with Grapefruit

◼

MAKES 4 SERVINGS

The citrusy flavor of grapefruit complements an oily fish like salmon.

2 medium red or pink grapefruit
1 teaspoon olive oil
2 scallions, chopped
2 large salmon steaks (about
  1½ pounds)

½ cup seasoned dry bread
  crumbs

Preheat the oven to 400 degrees F.

    Remove the peel and pith from the grapefruit. With a grapefruit knife, cut the segments free of the encasing membrane. Drain them. (The juice makes a refreshing drink for the cook.) Put the grapefruit in a pie pan, and sprinkle it with the oil and scallions.

    Wash and pat dry the salmon. Place the steaks in an oiled baking pan. Sprinkle them with the crumbs. Bake for 10 minutes on the top oven rack. Put the grapefruit in the oven and continue baking the fish until it flakes apart easily, 5 to 7 more minutes.

    Halve each salmon steak. Divide the salmon and grapefruit among 4 dinner plates.

Kilocalories 299 Kc • Protein 35 gm • Fat 12 gm • Percent of calories from fat 37% • Cholesterol 93 mg • Dietary fiber 2 gm • Sodium 97 mg • Calcium 44 mg

ANTIOXIDANT POWER

148

Fresh Salmon and Watercress Salad

■

Watercress yellows fast, but it will keep better if you treat it like a bunch of flowers. After rinsing the leaves, set the stems into a pitcher of water, cover the whole loosely with a plastic bag, and refrigerate until needed.

1 tablespoon olive oil
¼ cup chopped shallots
1½ pounds salmon fillets, with skin (1¼ pounds if skinned)

1 (8-ounce) bottle clam juice

For the vinaigrette

6 tablespoons unseasoned rice vinegar
2 tablespoons olive oil

1 teaspoon Dijon mustard
Freshly ground black pepper

1 bunch watercress
2 inner celery stalks with leaves, chopped
4 scallions, chopped

8 radishes, sliced
2 teaspoons drained capers

In a 12-inch skillet, heat 1 tablespoon of oil and sauté the shallots until softened, about 3 minutes. Place the salmon fillets on top and add the clam juice. Cover and cook at the lowest simmer until the salmon just flakes apart, about 8 minutes. Use a spatula to gently remove the salmon to a platter. Use a knife and fork to remove the skin and to separate the fish into large flakes. Chill the salmon.

To make the vinaigrette, whisk together the vinegar, olive oil, and mustard until well blended. Add black pepper to taste.

Wash the watercress, spin dry, and chop it into bite-size pieces, discarding the tough stems. Divide the greens among 4 chilled plates. Gently mix the salmon with the vegetables and vinaigrette, and spoon the mixture over the watercress. Sprinkle each serving with ½ teaspoon capers.

Kilocalories 343 Kc • Protein 35 gm • Fat 21 gm • Percent of calories from fat 58% • Cholesterol 93 mg • Dietary fiber 1 gm • Sodium 187 mg • Calcium 77 mg

Scallop Sauté on Steamed Broccoli de Rabe

MAKES 4 SERVINGS

Sea scallops are better for sautéing, because they'll turn a nice golden color instead of merely steaming. Bay scallops are cheaper and work fine for casseroles and pasta dishes.

1 bunch broccoli de rabe (about ¾ pound)

2 garlic cloves, chopped

3 tablespoons unbleached all-purpose flour

3 tablespoons cornmeal

1¼ pounds sea scallops, rinsed, extra-large scallops cut in half

3 tablespoons olive oil

½ cup mixed pitted chopped Sicilian green and Greek black olives

1 tablespoon drained capers

Juice of ½ lemon

Freshly ground black pepper

Wash the broccoli de rabe well, trim off the tough stems, and chop it coarsely. Boil 1 inch of water in the bottom of a steamer and put the broccoli de rabe in the steamer basket with 1 clove of chopped garlic. Steam until tender, about 10 minutes depending on the age of the broccoli de rabe. Keep it warm while cooking the scallops.

In a plastic bag, combine the flour and cornmeal. Add the scallops, hold the bag closed, and shake to coat. Shake off any excess coating.

In a 12-inch skillet, heat the oil until it's quite hot. Quickly stir-fry the scallops until they are golden and cooked through, about 5 minutes. Reduce the heat, let the pan cool a bit, then add the remaining clove of chopped garlic and sauté over low heat for 1 minute to cook the garlic. Stir in the olives and capers.

Arrange the broccoli de rabe on a platter. Remove the scallops, olives, and capers from the skillet and place them on top of the broccoli de rabe. Season the dish with lemon juice and black pepper to taste.

Kilocalories 301 Kc • Protein 30 gm • Fat 14 gm • Percent of calories from fat 39% • Cholesterol 60 mg • Dietary fiber 3 gm • Sodium 570 mg • Calcium 192 mg

ANTIOXIDANT POWER

150

Shrimp and Artichoke Stew

This provincial stew is full of delicious chunky ingredients in a golden broth that cries out for a crusty loaf of French bread. Just add a green salad and the menu is complete.

½ teaspoon saffron threads

2 cups vegetable stock (page 11) or canned low-sodium broth, warmed

2 tablespoons olive oil

¼ cup chopped shallots

1 red bell pepper, seeded and diced

1 cup diced fennel or celery

1 (8-ounce) bottle clam juice

3 medium red potatoes, scrubbed, cut into sixths

1 (9-ounce) package frozen artichoke hearts, separated (see Note)

4 strips lemon peel

1 teaspoon chopped fresh thyme or ¼ teaspoon dried

Salt (optional)

Freshly ground black pepper

2 tablespoons cornstarch

¼ cup cold water

1¼ pounds cooked shelled cleaned large shrimp (page 18 or use frozen cooked shrimp, thawed)

Crumble the saffron between your fingers and stir it into the warm vegetable broth. Let stand.

Heat the oil in a large pot, and slowly sauté the shallots, bell pepper, and fennel or celery until they are soft but not brown, 8 to 10 minutes. Add the vegetable broth, clam juice, potatoes, artichoke hearts, lemon peel, thyme, salt if needed (taste the broth), and pepper to taste. Bring to a boil and simmer, covered, until the potatoes and artichokes are tender, about 10 minutes.

Stir the cornstarch into the water until it's dissolved. Add to the simmering stew, and stir until it bubbles again and thickens slightly, about 1 minute. Simmer 2 to 3 minutes. Taste to correct the seasoning, adding salt if needed and pepper to taste. Add the shrimp and cook over very low heat for 1 minute.

Serve the stew in shallow soup bowls.

NOTE: The artichokes can be thawed enough to separate quickly by putting them in a strainer and running tepid water over them. The shrimp can be thawed the same way.

Kilocalories 331 Kc • Protein 34 gm • Fat 9 gm • Percent of calories from fat 24% • Cholesterol 277 mg • Dietary fiber 6 gm • Sodium 555 mg • Calcium 106 mg

RED SNAPPER AND ARTICHOKE STEW: Follow the preceding recipe, substituting 1½ pounds red snapper, cut into 2-inch chunks, for the shrimp. When the other ingredients are tender, add the fish, cover, and simmer until the chunks are cooked through, about 5 minutes.

Kilocalories 361 Kc • Protein 39 gm • Fat 10 gm • Percent of calories from fat 24% • Cholesterol 63 mg • Dietary fiber 6 gm • Sodium 347 mg • Calcium 105 mg

Shrimp and Avocado with Julienne Vegetables

■

MAKES 4 SERVINGS

This luncheon main dish or light summer supper suggests a new way for using broccoli stalks left over from recipes that call for florets only.

2 large carrots, cut in julienne
1 large broccoli stalk, peeled
  and cut in julienne
2 celery stalks, cut in julienne
½ red bell pepper, seeded and
  cut in julienne
2 large ripe avocados
2 tablespoons fresh lemon juice

1 pound cooked shelled cleaned
  shrimp (page 18 or use frozen,
  cooked shrimp thawed)
½ cup or more Dijon Honey
  Dressing (page 21)
1 tablespoon chopped fresh
  chives

Parboil the carrots and broccoli in boiling salted water for 1 minute, counting the time from when the water comes to a boil after adding the vegetables. Drain and rinse in cold water. When the vegetables are cool to the touch, toss them with the celery and bell pepper. Divide the vegetables among 4 plates.

Halve the avocados lengthwise. Pit and peel them. Place an avocado half on each "nest" of vegetables. Drizzle a little lemon juice over each avocado half.

Mix the shrimp with the dressing, adding more if needed, and spoon the shrimp over the avocado. Sprinkle with the chives.

Kilocalories 506 Kc • Protein 29 gm • Fat 37 gm • Percent of calories from fat 64% • Cholesterol 222 mg • Dietary fiber 9 gm • Sodium 340 mg • Calcium 122 mg

Shrimp and Cauliflower Salad

MAKES 4 SERVINGS

Keep the cauliflower crisp for this flavorful salad.

1 small head cauliflower (4 to 5 cups florets)
¼ cup mayonnaise
½ cup nonfat plain yogurt
1 tablespoon Dijon mustard
1 teaspoon chopped fresh dill or ¼ teaspoon dried

¼ teaspoon white pepper
1 pound cooked shelled cleaned shrimp (page 18 or use frozen, cooked shrimp thawed)
2 cups coarsely grated carrots (3 to 4)

Separate the cauliflower into florets; cut any large ones in half. Cook the cauliflower in boiling salted water until tender-crisp, about 3 minutes. Drain and rinse in cool water.

In a small bowl, blend the mayonnaise, yogurt, mustard, dill, and pepper.

In a large salad bowl, toss the shrimp and cauliflower with the dressing. Garnish with the grated carrots. Chill for at least an hour before serving.

Kilocalories 286 Kc • Protein 28 gm • Fat 13 gm • Percent of calories from fat 41% • Cholesterol 232 mg • Dietary fiber 5 gm • Sodium 409 mg • Calcium 141 mg

Seafood Casserole with Broccoli

---■---

MAKES 4 SERVINGS

Sherry in the sauce gives a Newburg flavor to this favorite fish dish. Although scrod is called for in the recipe, any filleted white fish could be substituted.

1 broccoli crown, cut into small
  florets and ½-inch-stalk slices
  (½ to ¾ pound)
3 red potatoes, peeled and
  sliced into ½-inch rounds
  (1½ pounds)
1 pound scrod
2 cups low-fat milk
½ teaspoon whole black
  peppercorns
¼ cup nonfat dry milk powder
3 tablespoons superfine flour,
  such as Wondra

¼ teaspoon salt
¼ teaspoon paprika
Dashes of cayenne to taste
3 tablespoons dry sherry
  (optional)
1 teaspoon soft butter
12 large cooked shelled cleaned
  shrimp (page 18)
1 cup fresh bread crumbs from
  1 slice Italian bread
¼ cup freshly grated Parmesan
  cheese

Cook the broccoli in boiling salted water until just tender-crisp, 3 minutes. Drain. In the same water, boil the potatoes until just tender, 5 minutes. Drain.

Put the scrod in a medium nonstick skillet with 1 cup milk and the peppercorns. Bring to a simmer, cover, and poach over very low heat until the fish is just cooked through, about 8 minutes. Gently remove the fish with a spatula, making sure no peppercorns are clinging to it.

Strain the milk, discarding the peppercorns. Put it into a medium saucepan. Whisk the dry milk, flour, salt, paprika, and cayenne into the remaining 1 cup cold liquid milk. Add this mixture to the milk in the saucepan, and cook over medium heat, stirring constantly, until bubbling and thickened, about 3 minutes. Add the sherry. Simmer over very low heat for 3 minutes, stirring often.

Preheat the oven to 350 degrees F.

Butter a 2½-quart gratin dish. Layer the potatoes on the bottom, then the broccoli. Add the fish in large flakes. Arrange the shrimp between the flakes. Pour the sauce over all. Sprinkle with the crumbs and cheese. Bake until browned and bubbling, about 20 minutes if the ingredients are still warm.

Kilocalories 427 Kc • Protein 46 gm • Fat 7 gm • Percent of calories from fat 15% • Cholesterol 175 mg • Dietary fiber 5 gm • Sodium 570 mg • Calcium 328 mg

Asparagus and
Vermicelli Frittata

‖

MAKES 6 SERVINGS

I often use a combination of eggs and egg substitute, a compromise that lowers the cholesterol without sacrificing flavor. If you don't have a cholesterol problem, the American Heart Association says it's okay to enjoy three to four eggs a week.

1 pound fresh asparagus (short
   spears are best)
4 ounces vermicelli
2 tablespoons olive oil
4 scallions, chopped
6 large eggs or 3 eggs plus
   ¾ cup prepared egg
   substitute, such as Egg
   Beaters

1 tablespoon minced fresh flat-
   leaf parsley
¼ teaspoon salt
⅛ teaspoon freshly ground black
   pepper
¼ cup freshly grated Parmesan
   cheese

Trim off the woody ends of the asparagus and wash the stalks well. Lay them in a large skillet with about ½ inch salted water. Bring to a boil, cover, and reduce the heat. Cook until tender-crisp, 2 to 3 minutes, depending on the thickness of the stalks. Drain and rinse in cold water (in the skillet is the easiest way) until the stalks are no longer warm. Drain again.

Cook the vermicelli according to package directions, drain, and mix with ½ tablespoon oil. Heat the remaining 1½ tablespoons oil in a 12-inch nonstick skillet and sauté the scallions until they are soft but not brown, about 2 minutes. Beat the eggs with the parsley, salt, and pepper.

Spoon the vermicelli into the skillet, spreading evenly. Lay the asparagus on top in a wheel-spoke pattern, tips toward the rim of the pan. Carefully pour the eggs over all and press the asparagus into the mixture slightly. Cook over low heat until the eggs have formed a crust, 5 to 7 minutes. While the eggs are setting, lift the frittata occasionally to allow any uncooked egg to run underneath.

Invert the frittata onto a 12-inch-round serving plate or platter, and slip it back into the pan to brown the second side, about 5 minutes. When ready, invert it again onto the plate in order to display the pretty asparagus pattern. Sprinkle with cheese and cut into 6 wedges to serve.

Kilocalories 218 Kc • Protein 12 gm • Fat 11 gm • Percent of calories from fat 47% • Cholesterol 215 mg • Dietary fiber 1 gm • Sodium 234 mg • Calcium 87 mg

Zucchini and Red Bell Pepper Frittata

■

MAKES 6 SERVINGS

6 large eggs or 3 eggs plus
  ¾ cup prepared egg substitute,
  such as Egg Beaters
1 tablespoon minced fresh flat-
  leaf parsley
¼ teaspoon salt
⅛ teaspoon freshly ground black
  pepper

2 tablespoons olive oil
1 small onion, chopped
1 red bell pepper, seeded
  and diced
1 small zucchini, sliced

Beat together the eggs, parsley, and seasonings. Heat the oil in a 12-inch nonstick skillet, and sauté the onion and bell pepper until they are tender and beginning to color, about 3 minutes. Push them to the sides and lay the zucchini slices over the bottom of the skillet. Continue to cook until the slices are tender, 2 to 3 minutes, then stir the bell pepper and onion gently into the zucchini.

Pour the eggs carefully over all. Cook over medium-low heat, lifting occasionally to allow the uncooked portion to flow underneath, until the eggs are set throughout, about 5 minutes. Carefully loosen the frittata and invert it onto a 12-inch serving plate or platter, then slip it back into the pan to brown the second side. Cut into 6 wedges to serve.

Kilocalories 129 Kc • Protein 7 gm • Fat 10 gm • Percent of calories from fat 67% • Cholesterol 212 mg • Dietary fiber 1 gm • Sodium 162 mg • Calcium 34 mg

Huevos Rancheros

It's a spicy "wake-up call"—with a carrot sneaking in some extra beta-carotene

2 tablespoons sunflower or any vegetable oil

1 medium yellow onion, chopped

1 green bell pepper, seeded and chopped

1 to 2 fresh or canned jalapeño chilies, seeded and minced (wear rubber gloves)

2 garlic cloves, minced

2 cups peeled chopped tomatoes, fresh ripe or canned drained (but still juicy)

1 large carrot, coarsely grated

1 teaspoon ground cumin

¼ teaspoon salt

4 eggs

½ cup coarsely grated Monterey Jack cheese

1 tablespoon minced fresh cilantro

4 slices whole wheat toast, halved diagonally

Heat the oil in a nonstick 10-inch skillet, and sauté the onion, bell pepper, and jalapeño until softened, 3 to 5 minutes. Add the garlic and sauté for 1 more minute. Add the tomatoes, carrot, cumin, and salt, and simmer the sauce, uncovered, stirring often, until the mixture reaches a sauce consistency but is not dried out, about 10 minutes.

Break 1 egg into a cup. Make a slight indentation in the sauce with the back of a cooking spoon, and carefully pour the egg into the simmering sauce. Do the same with the remaining eggs. Cover the pan and simmer over very low heat until the eggs are cooked through, about 4 minutes (the yolks can be partly runny, to your taste). Sprinkle the cheese and cilantro on top, remove from the heat, and cover the pan again for 1 minute to melt the cheese. Serve at once with hot toast triangles.

Kilocalories 348 Kc • Protein 17 gm • Fat 16 gm • Percent of calories from fat 40% • Cholesterol 217 mg • Dietary fiber 6 gm • Sodium 438 mg • Calcium 197 mg

ANTIOXIDANT POWER

Spicy Vegetable Gumbo

―――――――― ■ ――――――――

MAKES 4 SERVINGS

Making a real gumbo roux is time-consuming, but it can be made ahead and reheated when needed.

3 tablespoons canola oil
¼ cup unbleached all-
    purpose flour
2 Anaheim chilies, seeded
    and diced
1 large yellow onion, diced
1 celery stalk, diced
2 garlic cloves, minced
1 (14- to 16-ounce) can plum
    tomatoes with juice
⅓ pound fresh okra, trimmed
    and sliced
1 (16-ounce) can pinto beans,
    drained and rinsed

½ pound collard greens,
    chopped
1 teaspoon hot pepper sauce,
    such as Tabasco
½ teaspoon dried thyme
¼ teaspoon cayenne
⅛ teaspoon freshly ground black
    pepper
½ teaspoon salt
1½ cups shelled fresh or frozen
    corn kernels
3 cups hot cooked white rice

In a large heavy pot, blend the oil and flour. Cook over medium-low heat, stirring very often, until dark golden brown, 20 to 30 minutes. Be patient and don't rush this step or settle for a paler color. On the other hand, don't burn the mixture either.

Stir the chilies, onion, and celery into the roux, and cook over low heat until the vegetables begin to soften, 5 to 8 minutes. Add the garlic and cook 1 minute longer. Add the tomatoes, ½ cup water, the okra, beans, greens, hot pepper sauce, thyme, cayenne, black pepper, and salt. Simmer, covered, stirring often, for 20 to 25 minutes; the okra should be tender and the mixture thick and flavorful. Add the corn and cook 5 minutes longer. Taste to correct the seasoning, adding more salt or hot pepper sauce as desired.

Serve the gumbo in large soup plates with a spoonful of rice in the center.

Kilocalories 553 Kc • Protein 17 gm • Fat 12 gm • Percent of calories from fat 18% • Cholesterol 0 mg • Dietary fiber 16 gm • Sodium 337 mg • Calcium 146 mg

MAIN DISHES

Oven-cooked Vegetable Stew with Dumplings

MAKES 4 GENEROUS SERVINGS

Dumplings puff up better if you resist the impulse to lift the cover and peek at them while they're cooking.

2 tablespoons olive oil
1 large yellow onion, chopped
1 celery stalk with leaves, chopped
1 garlic clove, minced
2 carrots, sliced into 1-inch pieces
2 potatoes, peeled and cut into 2-inch chunks (¾ pound)
1 cup chopped canned tomatoes, undrained
3 cups vegetable stock (page 11) or canned low-sodium broth

¼ cup pearl barley, rinsed
¾ teaspoon salt
⅛ teaspoon freshly ground black pepper
2 cups fresh or frozen cut green beans
1 small zucchini, cut into 1-inch chunks
¼ cup pitted, sliced, or halved black olives
1 teaspoon chopped fresh rosemary or ¼ teaspoon dried

For the dumplings

1½ cups unbleached all-purpose flour
3½ teaspoons baking powder
¼ teaspoon salt

¼ teaspoon white pepper
2 tablespoons finely chopped fresh chives or flat-leaf parsley
About ¾ cup whole or 2% milk

Preheat the oven to 375 degrees F.

Heat the oil in a Dutch oven or large range-to-oven heavy casserole with a cover, and sauté the onion and celery until they are lightly colored, about 5 minutes. Add the garlic during the last minute.

Add the carrots, potatoes, tomatoes, stock, barley, ¼ teaspoon salt, and the black pepper. Bring to a boil on the range top. Cover and bake for 25 minutes.

Meanwhile, to make the dumplings, sift the flour with the baking powder, salt, and white pepper. Stir in the chives. Add enough milk to make a dough and stir with a fork until just blended.

Remove the dish from the oven and stir in the green beans, zucchini, olives, and rosemary. Bring to a boil. Remove from the heat and quickly drop the dumpling batter by heaping spoonfuls onto the stew (you should have about 8 dumplings). Cover and continue baking for 20 minutes, or until the dumplings are puffed and dry inside.

Kilocalories 459 Kc • Protein 13 gm • Fat 11 gm • Percent of calories from fat 20% • Cholesterol 6 mg • Dietary fiber 9 gm • Sodium 713 mg • Calcium 321 mg

Subgum Vegetables with Tofu

---■---

MAKES 4 SERVINGS

Tofu is well endowed with chemicals that ward off many forms of cancer.

1½ cups raw brown rice
⅓ cup vegetable or chicken
   stock (pages 11, 10) or canned
   low-sodium broth
1 tablespoon naturally brewed
   reduced-sodium soy sauce
2 tablespoons dry vermouth or
   dry sherry (optional)
½ teaspoon sugar
2 tablespoons or more
   peanut oil
1 pound firm tofu, diced
2 medium carrots, cut
   diagonally into very thin slices

1 green bell pepper, seeded and
   cut into triangles
2 celery stalks, cut diagonally
   into 2-inch pieces
1 medium red onion, peeled and
   cut into thin wedges
4 ounces fresh shiitake
   mushrooms, cleaned and
   sliced (discard the stems)
1 cup bean sprouts
1 (4-ounce) can water chestnuts,
   drained, cut into slices
1 tablespoon cornstarch

Cook the brown rice according to package directions.

Mix the stock, soy sauce, wine or sherry, if using, and sugar.

Heat the peanut oil in a large wok or skillet, and stir-fry the tofu, being careful not to break up the pieces, until lightly colored, about 3 minutes. Remove the tofu. Add more oil if needed and stir-fry the carrots for 2 minutes. Add the bell pepper, celery, onion, and mushrooms, and continue to stir-fry until the vegetables are tender-crisp, about 3 minutes. Add the bean sprouts and water chestnuts, and cook 1 minute longer.

Stir the cornstarch into the stock mixture until dissolved. Pour the sauce into the wok, and stir constantly until it thickens and glazes the vegetables, about 1 minute. Gently stir in the reserved tofu. Serve the vegetables with the rice.

Kilocalories 464 Kc • Protein 15 gm • Fat 10 gm • Percent of calories from fat 20% • Cholesterol 0 mg • Dietary fiber 8 gm • Sodium 289 mg • Calcium 100 mg

ANTIOXIDANT POWER

162

Italian Vegetable Stew

—■—

Serve the stew as a main dish with freshly cooked polenta (page 12) or with a loaf of crusty bread. Add a cool green salad on the side.

Salt

1 large eggplant, peeled and sliced (about 1 pound)

2 tablespoons olive oil

1 red bell pepper, seeded and cut into strips

1 green bell pepper, seeded and cut into strips

1 large yellow onion, chopped

2 cups drained canned tomatoes, chopped (most of a 28-ounce can)

2 large red potatoes, scrubbed, cut into ½-inch-thick rounds, peeled or unpeeled (about 1 pound)

1 large zucchini, cut into ½-inch-rounds (about ¾ pound)

1 tablespoon chopped fresh basil or ½ teaspoon dried

1 tablespoon chopped fresh flat-leaf parsley

Freshly ground black pepper

1 tablespoon balsamic vinegar

Salt the eggplant. Allow the slices to drain in a colander for a half hour. Rinse the slices and press them dry between paper towels. Cut the slices into quarters.

Heat the oil in a Dutch oven or other heavy pot, and sauté the bell peppers and onion until they begin to wilt, 3 minutes. Add the tomatoes and cook until they begin to soften, 5 minutes. Add the potatoes, cover, and simmer for 5 minutes. Add the eggplant, zucchini, basil, parsley, ½ teaspoon salt, and pepper to taste. Cover and simmer until all the vegetables are very tender but not mushy, 15 to 20 minutes more, stirring several times. Stir in the balsamic vinegar.

Kilocalories 247 Kc • Protein 9 gm • Fat 7 gm • Percent of calories from fat 25% • Cholesterol 0 mg • Dietary fiber 9 gm • Sodium 453 mg • Calcium 45 mg

ITALIAN VEGETABLE STEW WITH PORTOBELLO MUSHROOMS: This is a spicier, richer-flavored version. Follow the preceding recipe with these changes: Omit the onion. Add 2 large portobello mushroom caps, sliced, and 3 garlic cloves, minced, with the bell peppers. Substitute 1 tablespoon chopped fresh oregano or ½ teaspoon dried for the basil. Add a few dashes of hot red pepper flakes.

Kilocalories 246 Kc • Protein 10 gm • Fat 7 gm • Percent of calories from fat 25% • Cholesterol 0 mg • Dietary fiber 9 gm • Sodium 456 mg • Calcium 58 mg

ITALIAN VEGETABLE STEW WITH CHICKPEAS: Follow either of the preceding vegetable stew recipes. Add 1½ cups homemade chickpeas (page 16) or 1 (14- to 16-ounce) can low-sodium chickpeas, drained and rinsed, with the zucchini and eggplant.

MAKES **6** SERVINGS

Kilocalories 232 Kc • Protein 10 gm • Fat 6 gm • Percent of calories from fat 22% • Cholesterol 0 mg • Dietary fiber 9 gm • Sodium 305 mg • Calcium 50 mg

Spinach Pie with a Cabbage Crust

---■---

MAKES **6** SERVINGS

Cabbage makes a neat "crust" for vegetable pies!

About 8 large cabbage leaves
Olive oil
1 garlic clove, minced
2 (10-ounce) packages fresh or
   frozen leaf spinach
1 pound ricotta cheese (can be
   part-skim)
2 eggs, beaten
4 tablespoons grated Parmesan
   cheese

1 tablespoon minced fresh
   parsley
¼ teaspoon salt
¼ teaspoon white pepper
1½ cups tomato sauce (page 14
   or use store-bought sauce from
   a jar)

Remove the outer leaves of a large green cabbage by cutting them free at the core end. Parboil them in a large pot of boiling water, a few at a time, until they are pliable, about 2 minutes. Drain them on a paper towel. Line a well-oiled 10-inch pie pan with the leaves, cores toward the center. The leaves should overhang the pan by about 2 inches.

Using the same large pot, now emptied, combine the garlic and spinach, and cook the spinach in only the water that clings to its leaves after washing until it's wilted, 3 to 5 minutes. If using frozen spinach, follow the package directions. Drain very well, pressing out any excess moisture, and chop the spinach.

Preheat the oven to 350 degrees F.

Mix the ricotta, eggs, 2 tablespoons of the Parmesan cheese, parsley, salt, and pepper until well blended. Fold in the spinach. Spoon the filling into the cabbage leaf–lined pan. Sprinkle with the remaining 2 tablespoons Parmesan cheese. Fold the overhang over the filling. Brush the leaves with oil.

Bake in the middle of the oven until set, about 50 minutes. If the top gets too brown, lay a sheet of foil over the top, untucked. Let stand 10 minutes before serving. Spoon some tomato sauce over each portion.

Kilocalories 214 Kc • Protein 16 gm • Fat 12 gm • Percent of calories from fat 50% • Cholesterol 98 mg • Dietary fiber 5 gm • Sodium 425 mg • Calcium 381 mg

Cabbage Rolls with Pistachio Brown-and-Wild Rice

MAKES 4 SERVINGS

Butternut and Bell Pepper Chowder (page 66) would be a good starter to this entrée. Serve crusty rye bread on the side.

½ teaspoon salt
1 teaspoon vegetable oil
¾ cup raw brown rice
¼ cup wild rice
¼ cup pistachios
¼ cup golden raisins
1 tablespoon chopped fresh flat-leaf parsley
¼ teaspoon ground cinnamon

¼ teaspoon ground cumin
¼ teaspoon ground coriander
12 to 14 outer leaves of a very large head of cabbage (2½ pounds)
2 cups tomato sauce (page 14 or use store-bought sauce)
½ cup vegetable stock (page 11) or canned low-sodium broth

Bring 4 cups water to a boil in a large saucepan. Add the salt, oil, brown rice, and wild rice. Reduce the heat and cook at a high simmer until the two rices are tender but not mushy, about 40 minutes. Drain the rice. Stir in the nuts, raisins, parsley, cinnamon, cumin, and coriander.

Meanwhile, core a large head of cabbage and remove the outer leaves. Bring a large pot of salted water to a boil and parboil the leaves, a few at a time, until the rib end will bend slightly, about 2 minutes. Lay them out on paper towels to drain. It's wise to prepare a few extras in case of breakage.

Preheat the oven to 375 degrees F.

Put a scant ¼ cup rice stuffing in each leaf. Roll up from the rib end, folding in the sides, and place in a well-oiled gratin pan. (If necessary, secure the rolls with toothpicks.) Mix the tomato sauce and stock, and pour the mixture over the rolls. Cover with foil. Bake for 40 minutes. Remove the foil and bake 10 minutes longer. (If you have used toothpicks, remove them before serving.)

Kilocalories 412 Kc • Protein 11 gm • Fat 13 gm • Percent of calories from fat 27% • Cholesterol 0 mg • Dietary fiber 12 gm • Sodium 474 mg • Calcium 200 mg

ANTIOXIDANT POWER

166

Broccoli de Rabe and Potato Tian

---■---

MAKES 4 SERVINGS

When you're craving the comfort of a high-carbohydrate dish, this one offers a bonus of antioxidant-rich broccoli de rabe.

¼ cup nonfat dry milk powder

3 tablespoons superfine flour, such as Wondra

½ teaspoon salt

1½ cups low-fat milk

¼ teaspoon white pepper

3 tablespoons grated Romano cheese

3 tablespoons Basil Pesto (page 13 or from a jar)

12 ounces large egg bows

1 bunch broccoli de rabe (about ¾ pound)

2 large red potatoes, quartered lengthwise

1 garlic clove, chopped

½ cup cracker crumbs

In a medium saucepan, whisk the dry milk, flour, and salt into the liquid milk. Cook over medium-high heat, stirring constantly, until bubbling and thickened, 3 to 5 minutes. Simmer over very low heat for 3 minutes, stirring occasionally. Stir in the white pepper and 2 tablespoons of cheese. Remove from the heat and stir in the pesto.

Cook the egg bows according to package directions and drain them. Toss with the pesto cream.

Wash the broccoli de rabe well, trim off the tough stems, and chop it coarsely. Put the potatoes in a large pot with salted water to cover. Put the broccoli de rabe and garlic on top. Bring to a boil, reduce the heat, and simmer, covered, until the vegetables are tender, 10 to 12 minutes. Remove the broccoli de rabe with a slotted spoon. Remove the potatoes separately. Cut the potato quarters into slices.

In a large shallow baking dish, layer half the egg bows, the potatoes, the broccoli de rabe, and finish with the remaining egg bows. Sprinkle with cracker crumbs and the remaining tablespoon of cheese.

When ready to finish the dish, preheat the oven to 350 degrees F. Bake the tian until it's piping hot throughout and the top is golden, 15 to 20 minutes (or more if the dish has been refrigerated). Let rest 10 minutes. Cut into squares to serve.

Kilocalories 586 Kc • Protein 24 gm • Fat 11 gm • Percent of calories from fat 17% • Cholesterol 91 mg • Dietary fiber 5 gm • Sodium 478 mg • Calcium 380 mg

Quinoa and Vegetable Pilaf with Hazelnuts

◾

MAKES 4 SERVINGS

Because quinoa, an ancient Incan grain food, is so protein-rich, it makes a satisfying vegetarian main dish.

1½ cups quinoa
3 cups vegetable or chicken stock (pages 11, 10) or canned low-sodium broth
¼ teaspoon salt (optional— taste-test the stock)
1 tablespoon olive or canola oil
½ large red bell pepper, seeded and diced
1 medium zucchini, thinly sliced
About 2 cups broccoli florets, cut small

1 medium carrot, very thinly sliced
1 celery stalk, very thinly sliced
4 scallions, chopped
2 tablespoons slivered fresh basil or ½ teaspoon dried
2 garlic cloves, finely minced
½ cup chopped hazelnuts (available in many supermarkets)

Thoroughly rinse the quinoa in a strainer (the grain has a natural bitter coating that rinsing removes). Put the quinoa into a medium saucepan with the stock and salt, if using. Bring to a boil, reduce the heat, and simmer, covered, until all the water is absorbed, 12 to 15 minutes. When quinoa is cooked, the grains turn from white to transparent and the spiral-like germ unfurls from the grain.

In a large nonstick skillet, heat the oil and sauté the bell pepper, zucchini, broccoli, carrot, celery, and scallions until they are lightly colored and tender-crisp, 4 to 5 minutes. Add the basil and garlic during the last minute. Fluff the quinoa and stir it into the vegetable mixture. Transfer to a serving dish. Sprinkle with hazelnuts.

Kilocalories 420 Kc • Protein 13 gm • Fat 17 gm • Percent of calories from fat 34% • Cholesterol 0 mg • Dietary fiber 7 gm • Sodium 74 mg • Calcium 106 mg

Chilean Beans, Squash, and Corn

Ancient Native American farmers efficiently planted squash, beans, and corn in the same "hill" so that the bean vine could use the corn stalk for support and the ground-hugging squash would discourage weeds. The three still make a great combination, as in this tasty stew.

2 tablespoons olive oil
1 large yellow onion, chopped
1 tablespoon sweet paprika
1 garlic clove, minced
1½ cups peeled seeded chopped fresh or canned undrained plum tomatoes (see Note)
1 pound winter squash (any kind), peeled and cut into 1-inch pieces
2 teaspoons chopped fresh oregano or ½ teaspoon dried
¼ teaspoon salt
Freshly ground black pepper

½ cup vegetable or chicken stock (pages 11, 10) or canned low-sodium broth (optional)
1 cup fresh or frozen corn kernels
2 cups homemade cranberry beans (page 16) or 1 (15- to 16-ounce) can low-sodium cranberry beans, drained and rinsed
Hot pepper sauce, such as Tabasco

Heat the oil in a large pot and sauté the onion with the paprika for 3 minutes. Add the garlic and cook 1 minute longer. Add the tomatoes, squash, oregano, salt, and pepper to taste. Cover and cook over low heat until the squash is quite tender, 15 to 20 minutes. Check that the mixture does not become too dry; add stock or broth if needed.

Stir in the corn and beans and simmer for 5 minutes. Add hot pepper sauce to taste.

NOTE: If you use canned tomatoes, it's okay not to seed them.

Kilocalories 298 Kc • Protein 13 gm • Fat 8 gm • Percent of calories from fat 23% • Cholesterol 0 mg • Dietary fiber 14 gm • Sodium 167 mg • Calcium 100 mg

Pinto Bean, Barley, and Eggplant Stew

■

MAKES 4 SERVINGS

Keep the pan hot and stir-fry briskly to prevent the eggplant from absorbing too much oil.

Salt

1 large eggplant (about 1 pound)

½ cup pearl barley

2 tablespoons olive oil, plus
more if needed

1 large red bell pepper, seeded
and diced

2 garlic cloves, minced

1 (1-pound) can plum tomatoes
with juice

6 chopped fresh basil leaves or
½ teaspoon dried

2 chopped fresh thyme sprigs or
¼ teaspoon dried

⅛ teaspoon freshly ground black
pepper

2 cups homemade pinto beans
(page 16) or 1 (14- to
16-ounce) can low-sodium
pinto beans, drained and
rinsed.

Peel, slice, and salt the eggplant. Allow the slices to drain in a colander for a half hour. While they are draining, cook the barley in a large pot of boiling salted water until it is tender, about 35 minutes. Drain and fluff the barley.

Rinse the eggplant and press it dry between paper towels. Dice the slices. Heat the oil in a 12-inch nonstick skillet until it's quite hot, and stir-fry the eggplant and bell pepper until they begin to soften, about 5 minutes. Add the garlic during the last minute.

Add the tomatoes, basil, thyme, ¼ teaspoon salt, and pepper, and cook, covered, until the vegetables are tender, 10 to 15 minutes. Stir in the beans and cook 5 minutes longer. Stir in the barley and cook 2 minutes.

Kilocalories 345 Kc • Protein 13 gm • Fat 8 gm • Percent of calories from fat 20% • Cholesterol 0 mg • Dietary fiber 18 gm • Sodium 169 mg • Calcium 111 mg

Baked Rice-stuffed Tomatoes

This dish makes a beautiful vegetarian entrée. If you wish, garnish with sprigs of parsley and thinly sliced cucumber rounds. Bruschetta with Broccoli de Rabe (page 39) makes a delicious accompaniment.

8 medium ripe tomatoes

2 tablespoons olive oil

4 scallions, chopped

1 carrot, coarsely grated

1 garlic clove, minced

½ cup short-grain rice, such as arborio

About ¾ cup vegetable or chicken stock (pages 11, 10) or canned low-sodium broth

¼ teaspoon salt

⅛ teaspoon freshly ground black pepper

1 tablespoon chopped fresh flat-leaf parsley

2 tablespoons toasted pine nuts

¼ cup finely crumbled feta cheese

1 cup fresh bread crumbs from 1 slice crustless Italian bread

Slice off the top of each tomato. Spoon out the seeds and pulp into a strainer set over a bowl. Squeeze the pulp to obtain as much juice as possible. Turn the tomatoes upside down to drain while making the rice.

In a small saucepan, heat 1 tablespoon of the oil, and "sweat" the scallions, carrot, and garlic until they are soft but not brown, 5 minutes. Add the rice and stir to coat the grains with oil. Measure the strained tomato juice and add enough stock to make 1 cup. Add the stock, salt, and pepper to the rice, bring to a boil, cover, and simmer until all the liquid is absorbed, about 18 minutes. Stir in the parsley, pine nuts, and cheese.

Preheat the oven to 375 degrees F.

Arrange the tomatoes in a nonreactive baking dish that will hold them upright. Stuff them with the rice mixture. Press a layer of bread crumbs on top of each and drizzle the remaining tablespoon of oil over all. Bake until the tomatoes are just tender and the crumbs are brown, about 20 minutes.

Kilocalories 341 Kc • Protein 8 gm • Fat 17 gm • Percent of calories from fat 44% • Cholesterol 14 mg • Dietary fiber 4 gm • Sodium 397 mg • Calcium 113 mg

MAIN DISHES

Baked Mushroom-stuffed Golden Peppers

Choose boxy-shaped rather than long peppers for stuffing. I find yellow peppers to be much more easily digested than green, for those who are sensitive to such things.

1 pound assorted mushrooms, including a few shiitake
3 tablespoons olive oil
½ cup chopped shallots
1 tablespoon chopped fresh tarragon or ½ teaspoon dried
¼ teaspoon salt
Freshly ground black pepper
3 cups fresh bread crumbs from 3 slices Italian bread
¼ cup toasted wheat germ
½ cup freshly grated Parmesan cheese

1 tablespoon chopped fresh flat-leaf parsley
About 3 tablespoons stock or canned broth (any kind) or water
4 large yellow bell peppers, seeded and quartered lengthwise
1 (14- to 16-ounce) can chopped stewed tomatoes with juice

Preheat the oven to 375 degrees F.

Clean and slice the mushrooms; discard the stems on the shiitakes only. Heat the oil in a large nonstick skillet, and sauté the mushrooms and shallots over medium-high heat, stirring often, until their juices evaporate and they begin to brown, about 5 minutes. Season them with tarragon, salt, and pepper. Add the bread crumbs to the pan and sauté over low heat, stirring, until the crumbs are golden, about 1 minute. Remove from the heat, and stir in the wheat germ, cheese, and parsley. Add enough stock to make a moist but not mushy stuffing.

Stuff the pepper quarters, mounding the stuffing. Place the peppers in an oiled baking dish, pour the tomatoes over them, and bake for 35 to 40 minutes, until the peppers are tender.

Kilocalories 303 Kc • Protein 12 gm • Fat 15 gm • Percent of calories from fat 44% • Cholesterol 8 mg • Dietary fiber 6 gm • Sodium 483 mg • Calcium 205 mg

All-Vegetable Shepherd's Pie

This robust vegetarian entrée makes an attractive presentation as well.

4 large russet potatoes (1½ to 1¾ pounds), peeled and cut into uniform small chunks
1 tablespoon white vinegar
⅔ cup nonfat plain yogurt
1 tablespoon minced fresh chives or scallion tops
½ teaspoon salt
¼ teaspoon white pepper
2 tablespoons olive oil
1 medium yellow onion, chopped
2 medium carrots, sliced

2 cups chopped fresh broccoli
1 cup vegetable stock (page 11) or canned low-sodium broth
½ teaspoon dried basil or thyme
Freshly ground black pepper
1 cup shelled fresh or frozen peas
1 cup fresh or frozen corn kernels
1 tablespoon cornstarch
¼ cup cold water
½ cup dry bread crumbs
Paprika

Boil the potatoes in salted water to cover, to which you've added the vinegar, until they are quite tender, 5 to 7 minutes. Drain and dry the potatoes for a minute over low heat. Mash the potatoes. Whip in the yogurt, chives, ¼ teaspoon of the salt, and the white pepper.

Preheat the oven to 375 degrees F. Heat the oil in a 2½-quart Dutch oven or other heavy range-to-oven pan, and sauté the onion until it's yellowed, 3 to 5 minutes. Add the carrots, broccoli, stock, basil, remaining ¼ teaspoon salt, and black pepper to taste. Cover and cook until the carrots are almost tender, about 4 minutes. Add the peas and corn. Simmer, covered, 2 minutes longer. All the vegetables should be tender.

In a cup, dissolve the cornstarch in the cold water and add it all at once to the simmering broth. Stir until it thickens. Simmer, uncovered, for 2 minutes, stirring often.

Top the casserole with the potatoes. Sprinkle with the crumbs and paprika. Bake 20 to 25 minutes (longer if the dish is made ahead), or until the sauce is bubbly and the topping nicely browned.

Kilocalories 340 Kc • Protein 12 gm • Fat 8 gm • Percent of calories from fat 20% • Cholesterol 0 mg • Dietary fiber 9 gm • Sodium 565 mg • Calcium 149 mg

MAIN DISHES

VEGETABLE CHEESE 'N CHILIES SHEPHERD'S PIE: Follow the preceding recipe. Stir 1 cup coarsely grated Monterey Jack cheese into the mashed potatoes. Sauté 1 jalapeño chili, seeded and minced (wear rubber gloves), with the onion. Add 1½ teaspoons chili powder with the basil. Substitute pinto beans for the peas.

Kilocalories 435 Kc • Protein 24 gm • Fat 11 gm • Percent of calories from fat 21% • Cholesterol 10 mg • Dietary fiber 12 gm • Sodium 489 mg • Calcium 416 mg

Vegetable Goulash

MAKES 4 SERVINGS

Caraway rye bread makes a good accompaniment.

2 tablespoons olive oil
5 to 6 ounces mushrooms, sliced
1 large yellow onion, chopped
1 large celery stalk, chopped
1 large red bell pepper, cut into strips
1 garlic clove, minced
1 tablespoon paprika
2 cups vegetable stock (page 11) or canned low-sodium broth
2 tablespoons low-sodium tomato paste
2 large carrots, sliced
2 large potatoes, peeled and cut into 2-inch cubes (about 1 pound)

1 broccoli crown, cut into florets and ½-inch stalk slices (½ pound)
2½ tablespoons unbleached all-purpose flour
¼ teaspoon salt
⅛ teaspoon black pepper
⅛ teaspoon cayenne
⅓ cup reduced-fat sour cream
1 tablespoon minced fresh flat-leaf parsley

In a Dutch oven or large heavy flameproof pot, heat the oil and sauté the mushrooms until their juices evaporate and they begin to brown, about 5 minutes. Add the onion, celery, and bell pepper and continue to sauté until they are sizzling and fragrant, 3 minutes. Add the garlic and paprika and cook 1 minute longer.

Add 1½ cups of stock, the tomato paste, carrots, and potatoes. Cover and simmer 5 minutes. Add the broccoli to the goulash. Cover and simmer 3 minutes, or until all the vegetables are tender. Pour the remaining ½ cup stock into a jar with a tight lid. Add the flour, salt, black pepper, and cayenne. Cover and shake until a smooth paste is formed. Pour all at once into the simmering goulash, and stir until bubbling and thickened, 1 to 2 minutes. Simmer over very low heat for 3 minutes, stirring often. Taste to correct the seasoning.

Remove from the heat and stir in the sour cream and parsley.

Kilocalories 282 Kc • Protein 9 gm • Fat 10 gm • Percent of calories from fat 29% • Cholesterol 7 mg • Dietary fiber 8 gm • Sodium 230 mg • Calcium 96 mg

Vegetable and Brown Rice Paella

1¼ cups raw brown rice
1 cup vegetable stock (page 11)
 or canned low-sodium broth
½ teaspoon loosely packed
 saffron threads
½ pound fresh asparagus, cut
 diagonally into 1-inch pieces
2 large carrots, cut into 1-inch
 pieces
2 tablespoons olive oil

1 large red bell pepper, seeded
 and cut into strips
1 medium onion, chopped
2 garlic cloves, minced
1 cup homemade chickpeas
 (page 16) or canned low-
 sodium chickpeas, drained and
 rinsed
Herb Aioli (page 26)

Cook the brown rice according to package directions, but only to the al dente stage, since it will be subject to further cooking.

Heat the stock. Crumble the saffron and stir it into the stock. Let the mixture stand while continuing with the recipe.

Cook the asparagus in boiling salted water until tender-crisp, about 3 minutes; drain. Cook the carrots the same way, about 7 minutes; drain.

Preheat the oven to 375 degrees F.

In a large paella pan or skillet with flameproof handle, heat the oil and sauté the bell pepper and onion until tender-crisp, about 5 minutes. Add the garlic in the last minute. Stir in the rice, chickpeas, asparagus, and carrots. Pour the stock over all, blending all ingredients gently but thoroughly. Bake the paella, uncovered, for about 20 minutes, until piping hot throughout. Serve from the pan. Pass the Herb Aioli at the table as a topping for the paella.

Kilocalories 403 Kc • Protein 11 gm • Fat 10 gm • Percent of calories from fat 21% • Cholesterol 0 mg • Dietary fiber 9 gm • Sodium 31 mg • Calcium 74 mg

ANTIOXIDANT POWER

176

Vegetable-Chickpeas Hot Pot

Tossed Greens with Fennel (page 291) would be a cool companion.

2 tablespoons olive oil

1 large yellow onion, chopped

2 green bell peppers, cut into strips

2 large potatoes, cut into 2-inch strips

2 large carrots, sliced

4 small turnips, peeled and halved

2 cups homemade chickpeas (page 16) or 1 (14- to 16-ounce) can low-sodium chickpeas, drained and rinsed

2 tablespoons unbleached all-purpose flour

2 garlic cloves, minced

2 bay leaves

Leaves from 4-inch fresh rosemary sprig or ¼ teaspoon dried rosemary

¼ teaspoon salt

⅛ teaspoon freshly ground black pepper

¼ cup thick tomato sauce

About 2 cups vegetable stock (page 11) or canned low-sodium broth

Preheat the oven to 375 degrees F.

Heat the oil in a flameproof casserole and sauté the onion until lightly colored, 5 minutes. Add the bell peppers, potatoes, carrots, turnips, and chickpeas, and sauté for 5 minutes. Add the flour and garlic, and sauté 2 minutes. Add the bay leaves, rosemary, salt, pepper, tomato sauce, and enough stock to come up to the top layer. Bring to a boil, stirring gently the whole time.

Set the pot, covered and still simmering, in the middle of the oven. Cook until all the vegetables are tender, about 35 minutes. Remove the bay leaves. Taste to correct the seasoning.

Kilocalories 362 Kc • Protein 12 gm • Fat 10 gm • Percent of calories from fat 23% • Cholesterol 0 mg • Dietary fiber 12 gm • Sodium 216 mg • Calcium 89 mg

MAIN DISHES

Meatless Zucchini Moussaka

■

MAKES 4 SERVINGS

A delicate dish, this moussaka is very much like a soufflé and must be served promptly when it's ready.

2 large zucchini (2 to
  2½ pounds)
2 to 3 tablespoons olive oil
1 pound low-fat ricotta
  cheese
1 egg, beaten
1 tablespoon minced fresh flat-
  leaf parsley
¼ teaspoon white pepper
2 egg whites
Pinch of cream of tartar
2 tablespoons unsalted
  butter

2 tablespoons unbleached all-
  purpose flour
1½ cups low-fat milk
½ teaspoon salt
⅛ teaspoon ground nutmeg
1 cup tomato sauce (page 14
  or use store-bought sauce
  from a jar)
¼ cup freshly grated Parmesan
  cheese

Slice the zucchini ¼ inch thick. Heat 2 tablespoons of oil in a large skillet and fry the zucchini slices in batches until they are golden on both sides, 1 to 2 minutes per side. Add another tablespoon of oil if needed, but, in general, zucchini does not soak up oil the way eggplant does.

Mix the ricotta with the egg, parsley, and white pepper.

Beat the egg whites until foamy. Add the cream of tartar and continue beating until soft peaks form.

Preheat the oven to 350 degrees F.

Melt the butter in a saucepan. Stir in the flour and cook over low heat, stirring often, for 3 minutes. In another pan or the microwave, heat the milk to a simmer and add it all at once to the flour. Raise the heat to medium and stir constantly until the sauce bubbles and thickens, about 3 minutes. Add the salt and nutmeg. Fold the beaten egg whites into the hot sauce.

Assemble the moussaka in a ceramic or glass baking dish with a 2½-quart capacity. Arrange a third of the zucchini slices overlapping slightly to cover the bottom of the dish. Make layers as follows: all the ricotta, then another third of the zucchini, all the tomato sauce, and the remaining third of zucchini. Top with the white sauce and sprinkle with the cheese. Bake for 40 to 45 minutes, or until the top is golden and the ricotta is set. Serve at once.

Kilocalories 414 Kc • Protein 29 gm • Fat 24 gm • Percent of calories from fat 52% • Cholesterol 100 mg • Dietary fiber 4 gm • Sodium 777 mg • Calcium 774 mg

Vegetable and Fruit Side Dishes

"Something yellow, something green . . ." so goes the old adage about balancing the elements of a meal, and that's still sound and sensible nutritional advice. But for both good taste and good health, here are a few more thoughts about "balance."

A perfect meal needs variety, and variety in food begins with color. Serving all-green, all-red, or all-brown foods makes for an unappetizing spread that is probably one-sided nutritionally as well. Flavor follows appearance. The flavors of a meal should not be constantly repeated, such as pasta with tomato sauce accompanied by a tomato-laced salad, or a butternut squash soup followed by Pumpkin-Pecan Bread Pudding, or a dinner in which everything is napped in a creamy sauce from the soup to the dessert. There should be differences in temperature and texture also. Add a cool salad if the entrée and side dishes are hot. Include something crunchy like Carrot Slaw with Scallions if all the other dishes are soft and tender.

But a perfect meal also needs to be a complementary blending of flavors. A "sweet" entrée like Chicken, Sweet Potato, and Apricot Stew will blend better with Green Beans with Lemon and Allspice than with a bitter Sautéed Radicchio Salad. On the other hand, a brunch with jalapeño-spiked Huevos Rancheros goes better with savory corn bread than with sweet muffins.

There's a bonus to this menu "balancing act." When you balance foods, you're also balancing vitamins and minerals, and nutritionists continue to stress that a variety of foods offers the best overall nutrition. The vegetable and fruit side dishes in this chapter offer many possible combinations to help you plan not only perfect menus but also meals enriched with a medley of marvelous antioxidants.

Shopping and Storing Savvy

When you cook and serve an abundance of fresh produce, you want to buy the finest available and to know how to preserve the antioxidant goodness of the vegetables you've chosen. The following guide offers a few suggestions and tips to help you. But the best advice on shopping for fresh produce is always to buy the seasonal specials grown locally. They haven't lost any of their nutritional value by having been shipped from afar, they're at their peak of perfection, and their price is the most reasonable. Enjoy these vegetables while they last, and move on to others when the season changes. It's a healthful, pleasant way of living in tune with the cycle of the year and staying in touch with nature.

Artichokes and Asparagus

First of the spring vegetables, both artichokes and asparagus should have firm, green, tightly closed heads. Avoid waste in asparagus by choosing a bunch that needs the least trimming of woody ends. Treat asparagus as if it were a bunch of flowers; store the stems upright in 1 to 2 inches of water. Cover the top of the bunch with a perforated plastic bag and refrigerate. Enclose and refrigerate artichokes in a perforated plastic bag. Artichokes and asparagus are best used within a day but may be kept for up to 3 days.

Beans, Green

At the market, choose crisp unblemished young beans, avoiding the large, mature, tough ones. Keep the beans refrigerated in a perforated plastic bag and use them within a day or two of purchase. For a salad, you could cook them one day and serve them the next. Green beans are available all year, but their peak season is from May to October.

Beans, Shell

A late summer and early fall vegetable, fresh shell beans appear in decorative pods patterned with red and white. These pods should be firm, not limp, with no signs of mold. At home, simply bag the beans in a perforated plastic bag, refrigerate, and use them within a day or two.

Beets

Judge fresh beets by the condition of their greens, which should be unblemished and lively looking. Beet greens should be stored like other greens (see below) and cooked within a day or so. The bulb portions will keep 1 to 2 weeks in a refrigerator crisper. Beets are available periodically year-round.

Broccoli

Look for a bunch with a fresh smell and medium stalks that aren't too woody. The tops should be a purplish green with no sign of yellow flowering. Wrap broccoli in a dish towel enclosed in a plastic bag and it will keep in the refrigerator for 3 to 4 days. Although the peak seasons for broccoli are March to April and October, it's available year-round.

Carrots

Whether sold in a bunch or packaged in a deceptive orange bag, judge them by their tops, which should not look moldy, and by their crispness; they should resist bending. Carrots are good keepers—2 weeks or more—but they must be refrigerated and kept in perforated plastic bags so that they won't become limp.

Corn

Fresh corn is the glory of late summer and should be enjoyed to the fullest! Suit your own special taste for either sweet early corn or yellow mature corn, judging freshness by the condition of the stem end, which should be pale green and damp, not opaque and white. Plan to cook fresh corn on the day you buy it, as its sugar begins to convert to starch the moment it's harvested. Refrigerate the ears, unhusked, until ready to cook.

Greens of all varieties

In choosing greens, look for fresh-smelling, unwilted, unyellowed greens. Headed greens, such as cabbage, brussels sprouts, and lettuce, should not show any signs of rust at the core. Greens will keep better if you don't wash them until you're ready to use them. Wrap them in a dish towel, and store the bundle in a plastic bag in the refrigerator crisper. With this careful treatment, most greens will keep from 5 days to a week. Watercress, however, turns yellow quickly but will last longer if stored like asparagus (page 182). Cabbage keeps longer than the average, 10 days to 2 weeks.

Onions, Garlic, Leeks, and Scallions

In choosing onions and garlic, look for firm bulbs with no signs of sprouting. Since the green portion of leeks will be discarded, choose a bunch with more white bulbs than stems. The opposite is true of scallions, whose greens are a tasty addition to salads or used as a garnish. Onions and garlic will keep for several weeks in a cool, dry, dark place. Leeks and scallions, on the other hand, need refrigerating in perforated plastic bags. They will keep 5 days to a week.

Peas

Fresh peas have a very short season but are worth whatever effort they require. As with shell beans, judge peas by the condition of their pods. Avoid yellowing, split pods with overmature or sprouting peas. Try to use peas on the day of purchase, or failing that, on the very next day. Like corn, they lose their sweetness fast.

Peppers

Suit the shape of the pepper to your culinary purpose. Boxy ones are nice for stuffing; long, evenly shaped peppers are useful for broiling. Feel the surface, avoiding those with soft spots that may not be showing brown yet. Refrigerated in a perforated plastic bag, peppers will keep up to a week.

Potatoes, Sweet

Beware the woody-ended ones. Look for smooth, unblemished, well-shaped potatoes. They don't keep as well as white potatoes, so plan to use them within 3 days. Sweet potatoes, like white varieties, prefer a cool, dry storage place.

Potatoes, White

Avoid sprouting, soft, ill-smelling potatoes and any that have a greenish hue to their skins. Choose low-starch potatoes, such as red potatoes, for plain steamed or salads, and high-starch potatoes, such as russets, for mashing or baking. Never refrigerate or freeze potatoes. Keep them in a cool, dry, dark place. The ideal storage temperature is 45 to 50 degrees F. They should keep for 2 weeks or more.

Squash, Winter, and Pumpkins

In choosing these edible members of the gourd family, avoid damaged, puckered, or cracked skins and soft brown spots. These vegetables are excellent keepers that will remain fresh for a week at room temperature—longer when refrigerated.

Tomatoes

Winter tomatoes aren't worth buying, so load up on tomatoes when they're locally grown, sweet, and bursting with vitamin C. A little green skin at the stem end is a feature of farm-fresh tomatoes, which are much tastier than all-red pulpy hothouse tomatoes and also much cheaper. Store tomatoes at room temperature to preserve their flavor; fresh tomatoes will keep 3 to 4 days.

Turnips and Rutabagas

The smaller, the sweeter is the case with purple-topped turnips. Choose rutabagas, however, not by size but by the condition of their rind, much as you would choose winter squash. Refrigerate and use turnips within a day or so, before they lose their moisture. Rutabagas can be kept a week or more.

Zucchini and Summer Squash

Small is better (sweeter and less seedy) in these two summer varieties with edible skins. Refrigerate them in perforated plastic bags and cook them within 3 days.

Roasted Asparagus Parmesan

Simply elegant, this side dish will make any simple meal rather special.

1¼ pounds fresh asparagus, woody ends removed
½ teaspoon salt
2 tablespoons olive oil
2 garlic cloves, peeled and sliced
Freshly ground black pepper
½ cup freshly grated Parmesan cheese
1 tablespoon minced fresh flat-leaf parsley
Lemon wedges for garnish

Put the asparagus into a large skillet with 1 cup water and the salt, and bring it to a boil. Boil 1 minute, and immediately drain and rinse the asparagus in cold water. Drain again very well. Place the asparagus on a platter. Drizzle with the olive oil and put the garlic slices between the stalks. Season with pepper to taste. Allow the asparagus to marinate for a half hour or so, gently turning them through the oil and garlic from time to time.

Preheat the oven to 400 degrees F.

Oil a large flat baking pan. Lay the asparagus and garlic in the pan in one layer. Sprinkle with the cheese. Bake until the asparagus is tender, about 8 minutes. If you wish, remove the garlic. Arrange the asparagus on a platter, sprinkle with parsley, and garnish with lemon wedges.

Kilocalories 140 Kc • Protein 8 gm • Fat 11 gm • Percent of calories from fat 67% • Cholesterol 8 mg • Dietary fiber 2 gm • Sodium 498 mg • Calcium 160 mg

ANTIOXIDANT POWER

Green Beans with Roasted Scallions

The simple technique of roasting adds a savory flavor to plain vegetables.

2 bunches scallions, white parts
    cut diagonally into 1-inch
    pieces
2 tablespoons olive oil
2 tablespoons balsamic vinegar
1 pound fresh green beans, ends
    trimmed, cut diagonally into
    2-inch pieces

1 teaspoon chopped fresh thyme
    or ¼ teaspoon dried thyme
    leaves
Salt and freshly ground black
    pepper

Preheat the oven to 375 degrees F. Combine the scallions and oil in a glass pie pan, and toss to coat. Roast the scallions until golden and tender, 15 to 20 minutes. Drizzle them with the vinegar.

Cook the green beans in a large pot of salted water until tender, 5 to 7 minutes. Drain. Season with the thyme and salt and pepper to taste. Combine the scallions and green beans, and heat through if necessary.

Kilocalories 116 Kc • Protein 3 gm • Fat 7 gm • Percent of calories from fat 51% • Cholesterol 0 mg • Dietary fiber 4 gm • Sodium 8 mg • Calcium 71 mg

VEGETABLE AND FRUIT SIDE DISHES

Green Beans with Lemon and Allspice

Like black pepper, allspice has a lot more flavor when freshly ground from the dried berries, which can be bought in herb and specialty shops.

2 tablespoons olive oil
¼ cup chopped shallots
1 pound fresh green beans, ends
   trimmed, cut into 1-inch
   lengths
1 cup chicken stock (page 10) or
   canned low-sodium broth

1 teaspoon grated lemon zest
½ teaspoon allspice, preferably
   freshly ground
¼ teaspoon freshly ground black
   pepper

In a 10-inch skillet, heat the oil and sauté the shallots until they are sizzling and fragrant, 3 minutes. Add the green beans and stock; cover and simmer until the beans are tender, 5 to 8 minutes. Sprinkle with lemon rind, allspice, and pepper, stirring to blend well.

Kilocalories 111 Kc • Protein 3 gm • Fat 7 gm • Percent of calories from fat 56% • Cholesterol 0 mg • Dietary fiber 4 gm • Sodium 14 mg • Calcium 55 mg

Gingery Green Beans

This is a nicely spicy dish to serve with broiled chops or baked fish.

1 pound fresh green beans, ends trimmed, cut diagonally into 2-inch lengths
1 tablespoon olive oil
1 large garlic clove, minced
1 fresh or canned jalapeño chili, seeded and minced (wear rubber gloves)

2 slices fresh ginger, peeled and finely chopped
¾ cup orange juice
1 teaspoon grated orange zest
½ teaspoon ground cumin

Cook the green beans in boiling salted water until they're tender, 5 to 7 minutes. Drain and rinse in cold water to stop the cooking.

In a medium skillet, heat the oil and sauté the garlic, chili, and ginger for 3 minutes; do not allow the garlic to brown. Add the orange juice, zest, and cumin. Bring to a boil and simmer 2 minutes. When ready to serve, heat the green beans in the ginger sauce.

Kilocalories 97 Kc • Protein 3 gm • Fat 4 gm • Percent of calories from fat 33% • Cholesterol 0 mg • Dietary fiber 4 gm • Sodium 5 mg • Calcium 63 mg

VEGETABLE AND FRUIT SIDE DISHES

Blue Green Beans

Roman or Italian green beans are broader and flatter than regular green beans. Meaty yet tender, they combine well with hearty flavors, as in the recipe below, or with vinaigrette in a salad.

1 pound fresh Roman beans or
   regular green beans, ends
   trimmed, cut into 1-inch
   lengths
4 scallions, ends trimmed, cut
   into 1-inch lengths

1 cup chicken stock (page 10) or
   canned low-sodium broth
½ cup crumbled blue cheese
Freshly ground black pepper

Combine the beans, scallions, and stock in a saucepan. Simmer the beans in the stock until they are tender, 7 to 10 minutes (the thick Roman beans take more time than thin green beans). Remove from the heat. Sprinkle with the blue cheese and pepper to taste. Let stand, covered, until the cheese melts, 3 minutes.

Kilocalories 111 Kc • Protein 7 gm • Fat 5 gm • Percent of calories from fat 42% • Cholesterol 13 mg • Dietary fiber 4 gm • Sodium 250 mg • Calcium 146 mg

Basque Beans

■

This is a well-seasoned favorite from the north of Spain. Traditionally, diced or slivered ham or cooked sausage would be added, but this vegetarian version is also quite tasty.

1 pound fresh green beans, ends trimmed, cut into 1-inch pieces
2 tablespoons olive oil
1 hot dry red chili
2 garlic cloves, minced
2 cups peeled seeded chopped fresh tomatoes or 1 (1-pound) can Italian-style tomatoes, undrained
1 tablespoon minced fresh flat-leaf parsley
1 tablespoon chopped fresh basil or ½ teaspoon dried

1 tablespoon chopped fresh oregano or ½ teaspoon dried
1 teaspoon chopped fresh thyme or ¼ teaspoon dried
¼ teaspoon salt
¼ teaspoon freshly ground black pepper
2 cups homemade white kidney beans (cannellini) (page 16) or canned low-sodium beans, drained and rinsed

Cook the green beans in boiling salted water until tender-crisp, 5 to 7 minutes. Drain and rinse in cold water to stop the cooking.

In a 10-inch skillet, heat the oil and sauté the chili and garlic until they are sizzling and fragrant, 2 to 3 minutes. Add the tomatoes, parsley, basil, oregano, thyme, salt, and pepper. Simmer the sauce, uncovered, stirring often, until thickened, 20 to 25 minutes. Stir in the green beans and white kidney beans, and simmer to heat through and combine the flavors, 3 to 5 minutes. Remove the dried chili before serving.

Kilocalories 164 Kc • Protein 8 gm • Fat 5 gm • Percent of calories from fat 27% • Cholesterol 0 mg • Dietary fiber 9 gm • Sodium 111 mg • Calcium 84 mg

VEGETABLE AND FRUIT SIDE DISHES

191

Fresh Succotash with Tomatoes

---■---

MAKES 4 SERVINGS

This fresh version is much sweeter than the canned lima bean succotash of yesteryear.

2 tablespoons olive oil
1 large onion, chopped
1 mild green chili, seeded
  and diced
1 cup peeled seeded chopped
  fresh tomatoes
2 cups vegetable or chicken
  stock (pages 11, 10) or canned
  low-sodium broth
2 cups shelled shell beans
  (about 1½ pounds in the
  shells) or canned low-sodium
  shell or pinto beans, drained
  and rinsed

¼ teaspoon salt
2 cups fresh corn kernels, cut
  from the cob (about 4 ears)
2 teaspoons chopped
  fresh summer savory or
  ½ teaspoon dried
¼ cup chopped fresh chives
¼ teaspoon white pepper

In a large pot, heat the oil and sauté the onion and chili until lightly colored, 3 minutes. Add the tomatoes, stock, shell beans, and salt, and simmer the beans, covered, until they are tender, about 20 minutes. (If using canned beans, reduce the time to 8 minutes.)

Add the corn and savory, and simmer 5 minutes. Stir in the chives and white pepper. Keep warm 5 minutes before serving in bowls.

Kilocalories 297 Kc • Protein 12 gm • Fat 8 gm • Percent of calories from fat 23% • Cholesterol 0 mg • Dietary fiber 13 gm • Sodium 177 mg • Calcium 62 mg

Tuscan Beans

Although you must remember to soak dried beans the night before cooking them, they're very easy to make from scratch. These well-flavored beans make a spicy side dish or a hearty dressing for a pound of medium shell pasta.

1½ cups dried white kidney beans (cannellini)

1 onion, chopped

2 tablespoons olive oil

2 garlic cloves, finely chopped

1 cup tomato sauce (page 14 or use store-bought sauce from a jar)

1 tablespoon chopped fresh sage, 1 teaspoon dried sage leaves, or ½ teaspoon ground sage

½ or more teaspoon salt

¼ teaspoon freshly ground black pepper

A few dashes of hot red pepper flakes

2 tablespoons chopped fresh flat-leaf parsley

Spill the beans onto a tray, pick out any foreign material such as pebbles or twigs, and discard any shriveled beans. Rinse the beans thoroughly. Add 2 quarts of water and put the beans in a cool place to soak overnight. The next day, drain and rinse the beans, discarding the soaking water.

Add enough fresh water to measure about 2 inches above the beans, about 1 quart. Add the onion. Cook on a very low simmer until tender, about 1½ hours (much depends on the age of the beans), stirring occasionally, gently so as not to break the beans.

In a small skillet, heat the oil and sauté the garlic until it sizzles. Add the tomato sauce and sage; let the mixture stand while cooking the beans.

When the beans are tender, drain them. Add the tomato-sage mixture, salt, black pepper, and red pepper flakes to taste. Simmer 3 minutes. Stir in the parsley.

Kilocalories 217 Kc • Protein 12 gm • Fat 5 gm • Percent of calories from fat 21% • Cholesterol 0 mg • Dietary fiber 13 gm • Sodium 215 mg • Calcium 92 mg

VEGETABLE AND FRUIT SIDE DISHES

193

Black Beans and Yellow Rice

MAKES 4 SERVINGS

This South American favorite is a pleasing side dish to serve with chicken.

1 tablespoon olive oil
1 medium yellow onion, chopped
1 mild green chili, seeded and diced
½ red bell pepper, seeded and diced
2 cups vegetable or chicken stock (pages 11, 10) or low-sodium canned broth

½ teaspoon ground turmeric
½ teaspoon ground cumin
½ teaspoon ground coriander
1 cup long-grain rice
2 cups homemade black beans (page 16) or 1 (15- to 16-ounce) can low-sodium black beans, drained and rinsed

In a large saucepan, heat the oil and sauté the onion, chili, and bell pepper for 3 minutes. Add the stock, turmeric, cumin, and coriander, and bring the mixture to a boil. Stir in the rice, cover, and lower the heat. Let the rice simmer over low heat until all the liquid is absorbed, 15 to 20 minutes. Fluff the rice.

Heat the beans separately in a small saucepan. Stir the beans into the rice.

Kilocalories 365 Kc • Protein 12 gm • Fat 5 gm • Percent of calories from fat 11% • Cholesterol 0 mg • Dietary fiber 7 gm • Sodium 27 mg • Calcium 72 mg

ANTIOXIDANT POWER

194

Beets and Beet Greens with Fresh Herbs

MAKES 6 SERVINGS

Besides their high antioxidant content, beet greens are a good nondairy source of calcium. Beet greens are also high in natural sodium, so they need not be salted to be flavorful.

1 bunch beets with beet greens, separated
1 cup chicken or vegetable stock (pages 10, 11) or canned low-sodium broth—more, if needed
2 tablespoons olive oil

2 tablespoons fresh lemon juice
1 tablespoon chopped fresh dill
1 tablespoon chopped fresh chives or cilantro

Wash the beets and beet greens separately and well. Peel the beets and slice them ¼ inch thick. Chop the beet greens. Put the beets into a saucepan with the stock, bring to a simmer, and cook, covered, until they are nearly tender, 8 to 10 minutes. Add more stock if necessary. Add the greens and continue cooking until everything is tender, 5 to 8 minutes. Drain.

Put the vegetables into a serving dish and toss with the oil and lemon juice. Add the herbs and toss again.

Kilocalories 127 Kc • Protein 3 gm • Fat 5 gm • Percent of calories from fat 32% • Cholesterol 0 mg • Dietary fiber 6 gm • Sodium 190 mg • Calcium 58 mg

VEGETABLE AND FRUIT SIDE DISHES

Beet Greens in the Sicilian Style

Like many Sicilian dishes, this one is more flavorful when served at room temperature.

2 bunches beet greens (about
  1½ pounds)
2 garlic cloves, chopped
½ cup vegetable or chicken
  stock (pages 11, 10) or canned
  low-sodium broth

¼ cup dried currants
Freshly ground black pepper
2 tablespoons extra-virgin
  olive oil
1 tablespoon or more red wine
  vinegar

Wash the beet greens well and chop them coarsely. Combine the greens, garlic, stock, and currants in a large pot, cover, and simmer until the greens are tender, 5 to 8 minutes. Remove the vegetable with a slotted spoon to a serving dish. Season with pepper to taste. Toss with the oil and vinegar. Taste to determine if you want more vinegar.

Kilocalories 192 Kc • Protein 10 gm • Fat 8 gm • Percent of calories from fat 31% • Cholesterol 0 mg • Dietary fiber 11 gm • Sodium 879 mg • Calcium 424 mg

Sesame Broccoli

Sesame oil and sesame seeds, standards in Asian cooking, are great sources of vitamin E.

2 large broccoli crowns (1 to 1¼ pounds)
1 tablespoon peanut or any vegetable oil
1 teaspoon sesame oil
1 bunch scallions, cut into 1-inch pieces

2 tablespoons sesame seeds
1 tablespoon naturally brewed reduced-sodium soy sauce
Hot red pepper flakes

Cut the broccoli into ½-inch spears with the florets attached, about 4 cups loosely packed. Parboil the broccoli in boiling salted water until barely tender-crisp, about 2 minutes. Drain well and rinse in cold water to stop the cooking.

Heat the oils in a large skillet and stir-fry the scallions until tender-crisp, 2 minutes. Add the sesame seeds and cook 1 minute longer; don't over-brown the seeds. Add the broccoli and stir-fry 1 minute. Toss with the soy sauce and hot pepper flakes to taste. Turn out in a serving dish, which will put most of the sesame seeds on the top. Serve hot or at room temperature.

Kilocalories 103 Kc • Protein 5 gm • Fat 7 gm • Percent of calories from fat 55% • Cholesterol 0 mg • Dietary fiber 4 gm • Sodium 184 mg • Calcium 110 mg

VEGETABLE AND FRUIT SIDE DISHES

Broccoli and Butternut with Ginger Butter

MAKES 6 SERVINGS

Crystallized (candied) ginger is both sweet and hot. It's available in some supermarkets, in specialty stores, and occasionally in kitchen shops that stock herbs.

3 cups broccoli, florets cut small, stalks peeled and cut into ½-inch pieces

3 cups butternut squash, peeled and cut into 1-inch pieces (about ¾ pound)

½ teaspoon ground ginger

2 tablespoons unsalted butter, melted

2 tablespoons chopped crystallized ginger

Steam the broccoli until tender, about 5 minutes. Steam the squash until tender, about 8 minutes. Mix the ground ginger with the melted butter.

Combine the vegetables in a serving dish and toss with the ginger butter and chopped crystallized ginger.

Kilocalories 86 Kc • Protein 2 gm • Fat 4 gm • Percent of calories from fat 41% • Cholesterol 11 mg • Dietary fiber 2 gm • Sodium 58 mg • Calcium 51 mg

Brussels Sprouts with a Dutch Touch

Although fresh brussels sprouts are the best, when they're not available, frozen sprouts are a good product and can be substituted, except in stir-fries.

1 pound fresh brussels sprouts
1 tablespoon unsalted butter,
  cut into pieces
¼ cup low-sodium vegetable or
  chicken broth

½ cup finely diced Gouda cheese
¼ teaspoon caraway seeds

Trim the sprouts and cut an X in the core of each. Cook the sprouts in a large pot of boiling water until they are tender, 8 to 12 minutes. Drain. (Alternatively, prepare a 1-pound bag of frozen sprouts according to package directions, but undercook them slightly.)

Preheat the oven to 350 degrees F. Put the sprouts into a large gratin dish. Stir in the butter until melted. Pour the stock over the sprouts. Sprinkle with the cheese and caraway seeds. Bake until the sprouts are piping hot and the cheese has melted, 10 to 15 minutes.

Kilocalories 190 Kc • Protein 12 gm • Fat 12 gm • Percent of calories from fat 54% • Cholesterol 44 mg • Dietary fiber 5 gm • Sodium 319 mg • Calcium 268 mg

VEGETABLE AND FRUIT SIDE DISHES

Lemon-Poppy Sautéed Brussels Sprouts

MAKES 4 SERVINGS

To preserve the brightness of green vegetables, don't add lemon juice until just before serving.

1 pound fresh brussels sprouts	**Freshly ground black pepper**
1 tablespoon unsalted butter	**Juice of ½ lemon (about**
1 tablespoon olive oil	**2 tablespoons)**
1 large shallot, chopped	**2 teaspoons poppy seeds**

Trim the sprouts and cut an X in the core of each. Cook the sprouts in a large pot of boiling water until they are tender, 8 to 12 minutes. Drain. Rinse them in cold water and cut them in half through the base.

When ready to serve, heat the butter and oil in a large skillet and sauté the shallot until it's soft, 2 to 3 minutes. Add the sprouts and sauté until they are heated through, 1 to 2 minutes. Season with pepper to taste, lemon juice, and poppy seeds. Toss well before spooning into a serving dish.

Kilocalories 120 Kc • Protein 5 gm • Fat 8 gm • Percent of calories from fat 51% • Cholesterol 8 mg • Dietary fiber 5 gm • Sodium 60 mg • Calcium 83 mg

Brussels Sprouts with Dill and Celery Seed

The double celery flavor is especially savory, since celery contains quite a bit of natural salt. Fresh dill is best in this recipe.

1 pound fresh brussels sprouts
2 tablespoons vegetable oil
1 cup finely diced celery
½ teaspoon celery seeds

1 tablespoon chopped fresh dill
  or 1 teaspoon dried
Freshly ground black pepper

Trim the sprouts and cut a small X in the core of each. Cook the sprouts in a large pot of boiling salted water until they are tender, 8 to 12 minutes. Drain and rinse in cool water. Cut the sprouts in half.

Heat the oil in a 10-inch nonstick skillet and sauté the celery until tender-crisp, 5 minutes. Stir in the celery seeds and dill. Add the sprouts and warm them with the celery mixture to combine the flavors. Season with pepper to taste.

Kilocalories 115 Kc • Protein 4 gm • Fat 7 gm • Percent of calories from fat 51% • Cholesterol 0 mg • Dietary fiber 5 gm • Sodium 55 mg • Calcium 65 mg

VEGETABLE AND FRUIT SIDE DISHES

Braised Brussels Sprouts and Carrots with Balsamic Vinegar

───

MAKES 4 SERVINGS

1 pint fresh brussels sprouts
2 large carrots
1 tablespoon olive oil
1 large shallot, sliced

Salt and freshly ground black
  pepper
2 tablespoons balsamic vinegar

Trim the sprouts and cut an X in the core of each. Cut the carrots into ½-inch pieces. Parboil the sprouts and carrots in boiling salted water for 5 minutes. Drain.

   Heat the oil in a large skillet and sauté the shallot until it sizzles, about 1 minute. Add the drained vegetables and sauté, turning frequently, until they are lightly browned and tender, about 5 minutes. Season with salt and pepper to taste. Sprinkle with the vinegar.

Kilocalories 99 Kc • Protein 4 gm • Fat 4 gm • Percent of calories from fat 31% • Cholesterol 0 mg • Dietary fiber 5 gm • Sodium 39 mg • Calcium 53 mg

Brussels Sprouts and Carrots with Dijon Butter

───

MAKES 6 SERVINGS

The assertive flavor of brussels sprouts is complemented by flavorful Dijon mustard.

1 pound fresh brussels sprouts
½ pound carrots
3 tablespoons unsalted butter,
  melted

1½ tablespoons Dijon mustard

Trim the sprouts and cut an X in the core of each. Cut the carrots diagonally into ½-inch slices. Cook the sprouts and carrots in boiling salted water until tender, 8 to 12 minutes. Drain.

With a fork, whisk the butter into the mustard. Toss the mustard mixture with the vegetables.

Kilocalories 107 Kc • Protein 3 gm • Fat 7 gm • Percent of calories from fat 51% • Cholesterol 16 mg • Dietary fiber 4 gm • Sodium 115 mg • Calcium 49 mg

Stir-fried Chinese Cabbage

MAKES 4 SERVINGS

The secret to enjoying delicate cabbage dishes is to cook them quickly. Long cooking gives cabbage a strong flavor.

1 tablespoon peanut oil, or more if needed	1 tablespoon naturally brewed sodium-reduced soy sauce
1 large onion, thinly sliced	¼ cup dry vermouth or sherry
2 slices fresh ginger, minced	¼ cup low-sodium vegetable or chicken broth
1 garlic clove, minced	1 teaspoon cornstarch
1 pound Chinese cabbage, shredded (about 4 cups)	1 teaspoon sugar

In a large wok or skillet, heat the oil and stir-fry the onion, ginger, and garlic until the onion begins to soften, 2 minutes. Remove with a slotted spoon. Add more oil if necessary. Stir-fry the cabbage until it's just wilted, 3 minutes. Return the onion mixture to the wok.

Mix together the soy sauce, vermouth, and stock. Stir in the cornstarch and sugar. Pour over the vegetables, and cook over medium-high heat, stirring and tossing constantly, until the liquid thickens and forms a glaze, 1 to 2 minutes. Serve at once.

Kilocalories 93 Kc • Protein 3 gm • Fat 4 gm • Percent of calories from fat 35% • Cholesterol 0 mg • Dietary fiber 1 gm • Sodium 176 mg • Calcium 107 mg

Red Cabbage with Fried Apples

---■---

MAKES 4 SERVINGS

Serve this sweet-and-sour side dish with roasted chicken or pork.

2 tablespoons unsalted butter
2 Granny Smith apples, peeled, cored, and sliced
Cinnamon sugar for sprinkling (1 part cinnamon to 3 parts sugar)

4 cups shredded red cabbage
1 cup apple cider or apple juice
1 cinnamon stick
2 teaspoons cornstarch
1 tablespoon cider vinegar

Heat the butter in a large nonstick skillet, and sauté the apple slices until they are tender and lightly colored, 3 to 5 minutes. Sprinkle them with cinnamon sugar. Remove them from the skillet.

Put the cabbage, ¾ cup cider, and the cinnamon stick in the skillet, cover, and simmer until the cabbage is tender, 8 to 10 minutes. Remove the cinnamon stick.

Blend the cornstarch into the remaining ¼ cup cider and add it all at once to the cabbage. Cook over medium-high heat, stirring constantly, until the mixture bubbles and thickens, about 2 minutes. Stir in the vinegar. Simmer 1 to 3 minutes longer. Stir in the apples. Keep warm for 5 minutes or so before serving to blend the flavors. Taste to correct the seasoning. You may want to add more vinegar.

Kilocalories 127 Kc • Protein 2 gm • Fat 6 gm • Percent of calories from fat 45% • Cholesterol 16 mg • Dietary fiber 4 gm • Sodium 85 mg • Calcium 39 mg

Apple Cider Carrots

Some supermarkets sell one-pound bags of baby carrots, a great convenience.

1 pound baby carrots	1 tablespoon unsalted butter
1 cup apple cider	¼ teaspoon ground cinnamon
1 tablespoon honey	

Combine the carrots, cider, honey, butter, and cinnamon in a saucepan. Bring to a simmer and cook, covered, until the carrots are tender, 15 to 18 minutes. Remove the cover. Cook over medium-high heat, stirring often and watching carefully, until the juices are reduced to a syrupy glaze, 3 to 5 minutes.

Kilocalories 81 Kc • Protein 1 gm • Fat 2 gm • Percent of calories from fat 24% • Cholesterol 5 mg • Dietary fiber 2 gm • Sodium 62 mg • Calcium 22 mg

Honeyed Carrots

MAKES 6 SERVINGS

Cooking pan juices down to a glaze is a tricky business, but it gives carrots an especially sweet flavor.

1 tablespoon olive oil
2 large shallots, chopped
2 slices fresh ginger, minced
1½ pounds carrots, sliced
   diagonally into 2-inch pieces

2 tablespoons honey
¾ cup chicken stock (page 10)
   or canned low-sodium broth
Several dashes of white pepper

In a medium saucepan, heat the oil and sauté the shallots and ginger until sizzling, 1 to 2 minutes. Add the carrots, honey, and stock. Bring to a boil, reduce the heat, and simmer, uncovered, until the carrots are tender, about 8 minutes. Stir often and watch closely that the liquid cooks down to a glaze but does not boil out. Season with white pepper to taste.

Kilocalories 97 Kc • Protein 2 gm • Fat 3 gm • Percent of calories from fat 23% • Cholesterol 0 mg • Dietary fiber 3 gm • Sodium 46 mg • Calcium 31 mg

ANTIOXIDANT POWER

Carrots with Lemon and Cilantro

Cilantro also goes by the names of Chinese parsley or fresh coriander. It looks like flat-leaf parsley but has a much more pungent flavor, a favorite in Mexican, Indian, and Chinese cuisines. Dried cilantro has much less flavor, so use fresh if available.

1 tablespoon olive oil
1 garlic clove, chopped
1 pound carrots, cut diagonally
** into 2-inch pieces**
¼ teaspoon salt

2 tablespoons or more fresh
** lemon juice**
Freshly ground black pepper
1 tablespoon minced fresh
** cilantro or 1 teaspoon dried**

In a medium saucepan, heat the oil and sauté the garlic until sizzling, about 1 minute. Add the carrots and turn to coat with the oil. Add ⅓ cup water and the salt, bring to a simmer, and cook, covered, until the carrots are tender, about 8 minutes, taking care that the water does not boil out. If any liquid remains, turn up the heat to high and cook, uncovered, watching and stirring constantly, until it evaporates. This tricky step adds a lovely sheen and flavor to the carrots.

Season with lemon juice and pepper to taste. Stir in the cilantro.

Kilocalories 55 Kc • Protein 1 gm • Fat 2 gm • Percent of calories from fat 37% • Cholesterol 0 mg • Dietary fiber 2 gm • Sodium 124 mg • Calcium 23 mg

VEGETABLE AND FRUIT SIDE DISHES

Carrots with Black Olives

To pit olives, whack them, a few at a time, with the flat side of a chef's knife, taking care not to let them fly off the cutting board. The pits can then be easily removed.

1 tablespoon olive oil
¼ cup chopped shallots
1 pound carrots, cut diagonally into 1-inch pieces
1 cup chicken or vegetable stock (pages 10, 11) or canned low-sodium broth

⅓ cup kalamata olives, pitted and halved
1 tablespoon minced fresh flat-leaf parsley

In a saucepan, heat the oil and sauté the shallots until they are sizzling and fragrant, 1 to 2 minutes. Add the carrots and stock. Cover and simmer until the carrots are tender, about 8 minutes. Remove the carrots with a slotted spoon and keep them warm.

Reduce any liquid in the pan to 2 tablespoons by fast boiling. Pour the reduced liquid over the carrots and toss with the olives. Sprinkle with the parsley.

Kilocalories 73 Kc • Protein 1 gm • Fat 3 gm • Percent of calories from fat 44% • Cholesterol 0 mg • Dietary fiber 2 gm • Sodium 227 mg • Calcium 21 mg

Carrots and Peas with Fresh Herbs

The best way to have fresh herbs at your fingertips is to create a window-sill garden in the kitchen. A grow lamp can make up for a less-than-sunny exposure.

1 tablespoon unsalted butter
1 garlic clove, minced
4 medium carrots, cut diagonally into ½-inch pieces
¼ cup low-sodium chicken or vegetable broth
2 cups shelled fresh or frozen peas

2 tablespoons fresh lemon juice
¼ teaspoon grated lemon zest
Freshly ground black pepper
1 tablespoon chopped fresh chives
1 tablespoon chopped fresh basil
1 teaspoon chopped fresh mint

In a large skillet, heat the butter and sauté the garlic until softened but not brown, about 2 minutes. Add the carrots and broth, cover, and simmer until almost tender, about 5 minutes. Add the peas and continue cooking for 3 minutes, or until both vegetables are tender. Watch carefully that the liquid does not boil out.

Blend the lemon juice and zest into the vegetables, distributing the zest well throughout. Season with pepper to taste and toss with the herbs.

Kilocalories 73 Kc • Protein 3 gm • Fat 2 gm • Percent of calories from fat 25% • Cholesterol 6 mg • Dietary fiber 4 gm • Sodium 139 mg • Calcium 17 mg

VEGETABLE AND FRUIT SIDE DISHES

Carrots and Green Beans with Mortadella

---■---

MAKES 4 SERVINGS

A little mortadella adds a big flavor to this great vegetable side dish.

1 tablespoon olive oil
1 small yellow onion, chopped
2 ounces mortadella, diced
2 large carrots, sliced diagonally
  into 1-inch pieces
½ cup or more chicken stock
  (page 10) or canned low-
  sodium broth

½ pound fresh green beans,
  ends trimmed, sliced into
  1-inch pieces
Freshly ground black pepper

In a 10-inch skillet, heat the oil and sauté the onion and mortadella for 3 to 5 minutes. Add the carrots and broth. Cover and cook 5 minutes, checking that the broth does not boil out. Add more as needed. Add the green beans and continue cooking until both vegetables are tender, about 5 minutes more. Season with pepper to taste.

Kilocalories 126 Kc • Protein 4 gm • Fat 7 gm • Percent of calories from fat 51% • Cholesterol 8 mg • Dietary fiber 3 gm • Sodium 197 mg • Calcium 44 mg

Curried Cauliflower and Carrots

■

A bay leaf added to the boiling water dispels some of that strong cauli-flower aroma. It also adds its own flavor to the vegetable, so use it only when it suits the recipe's flavor combination.

1 bay leaf

1 medium head cauliflower, separated into florets

3 medium carrots, cut diagonally into 1-inch slices

1 tablespoon unsalted butter

1 tablespoon olive oil

2 teaspoons mild curry powder

¼ cup low-sodium vegetable or chicken broth

Freshly ground black pepper

In a large pot of boiling salted water to which you've added a bay leaf, cook the cauliflower until tender-crisp, about 3 minutes. Remove with a slotted spoon. In the same water, cook the carrots until they are tender, 5 to 8 minutes. Drain.

In the same pot (rinsed and dried), heat the butter and oil. Add the curry and stir until well blended. Add the stock and let it boil to reduce by half, about 1 minute. Add the cooked vegetables and gently toss to coat them with the curry. Add pepper to taste.

Kilocalories 76 Kc • Protein 2 gm • Fat 5 gm • Percent of calories from fat 52% • Cholesterol 5 mg • Dietary fiber 4 gm • Sodium 48 mg • Calcium 27 mg

VEGETABLE AND FRUIT SIDE DISHES

Cauliflower with Fried Peppers

---■---

MAKES 6 SERVINGS

To retain cauliflower's pure white color, add vinegar to the cooking water.

1 medium head cauliflower,
    separated into florets (cut large
    florets in half)
1 tablespoon white vinegar
1 bay leaf
2 tablespoons olive oil
2 Italian frying peppers, seeded
    and diced

1 garlic clove, minced
1 tablespoon minced fresh flat-
    leaf parsley
Salt and freshly ground black
    pepper
Shaved Parmesan or Asiago
    cheese as a garnish (optional)

Cook the cauliflower in boiling salted water to which you've added white vinegar and a bay leaf until tender-crisp, about 3 minutes. Drain.

Heat the oil in a large skillet, and sauté the peppers until they are tender and lightly colored, about 5 minutes. Add the garlic during the last minute.

Stir in the cauliflower, add the parsley, and season with salt and pepper to taste. Toss gently but well to blend the ingredients. Transfer to a large serving dish and garnish with the shaved cheese, if desired.

Kilocalories 70 Kc • Protein 2 gm • Fat 5 gm • Percent of calories from fat 57% • Cholesterol 0 mg • Dietary fiber 3 gm • Sodium 15 mg • Calcium 20 mg

Gratin of Cauliflower and Tomatoes

—■—

This pretty casserole could be a vegetarian main dish. Green salad, brown rice, and corn bread might round out the menu.

1 small head cauliflower, separated into florets
1 tablespoon white vinegar
1 bay leaf
1 tablespoon olive oil
4 scallions, chopped
2 medium ripe tomatoes, cut into wedges
1 teaspoon minced fresh basil or ¼ teaspoon dried
Freshly ground black pepper
¼ cup seasoned bread crumbs
¾ cup coarsely grated Gruyère cheese

Preheat the oven to 350 degrees F.

Cook the cauliflower in boiling salted water to which you've added vinegar and a bay leaf until tender-crisp, about 3 minutes. Drain.

Combine the oil and scallions in a medium gratin pan or baking dish that will hold the cauliflower more or less in one layer. Put the scallions in the oven until they begin to sizzle, 3 to 5 minutes. Remove the pan and arrange the cauliflower in a layer with the tomato wedges tucked between the florets. Season with basil and pepper to taste. Sprinkle with the bread crumbs and cheese. Cover with foil.

Bake for 15 minutes. Uncover and continue baking until the tomatoes are cooked and the cheese has melted, about 5 more minutes.

Kilocalories 146 Kc • Protein 11 gm • Fat 8 gm • Percent of calories from fat 47% • Cholesterol 13 mg • Dietary fiber 4 gm • Sodium 81 mg • Calcium 234 mg

VEGETABLE AND FRUIT SIDE DISHES

Cauliflower in Lemon Cream

MAKES 6 SERVINGS

Like cabbage, cauliflower is much sweeter when not overcooked.

1 medium head cauliflower, separated into florets (cut large florets in half)
1 tablespoon white vinegar
2 tablespoons olive oil
2 tablespoons lemon juice

1 garlic clove, crushed through a press
Salt and white pepper
½ cup nonfat plain yogurt
1 teaspoon Dijon mustard
1 teaspoon grated lemon zest

Cook the cauliflower in boiling salted water to which you've added white vinegar until tender-crisp, about 3 minutes. Drain.

Mix together the olive oil, lemon juice, and garlic. Transfer the cauliflower to a bowl and toss with the dressing. Season with salt and white pepper to taste.

Mix together the yogurt, mustard, and grated lemon zest. Add this to the cauliflower and toss again. Serve warm or at room temperature.

Kilocalories 73 Kc • Protein 3 gm • Fat 5 gm • Percent of calories from fat 56% • Cholesterol 0 mg • Dietary fiber 2 gm • Sodium 31 mg • Calcium 54 mg

Cauliflower and Potato Casserole

—■—

This is just the right dish to make when you have leftover mashed pota-toes. Frozen cauliflower tends to be soft and watery, but it can be used for casseroles like this and for pureed soups.

2 tablespoons unsalted butter
1 small onion, chopped
2 cups mashed whipped
  potatoes
2 cups well-cooked mashed
  cauliflower (1 [10-ounce]
  package frozen cauliflower,
  cooked, can be used)

2 eggs, beaten, or ½ cup
  prepared egg substitute
⅛ teaspoon salt
⅛ teaspoon white pepper
5 tablespoons grated Romano
  cheese

Preheat the oven to 350 degrees F. Heat the butter in a small skillet and sauté the onion until it's limp and yellowed, 3 to 5 minutes; cool slightly.

Blend together the potatoes, cauliflower, onion, eggs, salt, pepper, and 3 tablespoons of the cheese. Spoon the mixture into a buttered 1½-quart casserole, and sprinkle the remaining 2 tablespoons of cheese on top. Bake in the middle of the oven until golden and piping hot, 30 to 35 minutes.

Kilocalories 227 Kc • Protein 10 gm • Fat 8 gm • Percent of calories from fat 30% • Cholesterol 118 mg • Dietary fiber 5 gm • Sodium 241 mg • Calcium 125 mg

Creamed Cauliflower

■

This versatile favorite has many tasty versions. In this recipe, it's a side dish, but creamed cauliflower can be turned into a vegetarian main dish simply by tossing it with a half pound of cooked pasta—medium shells are a perfect shape.

1 medium head cauliflower,
  separated into florets (cut large
  florets in half)
1 tablespoon white vinegar
1 tablespoon unsalted butter
1 shallot, minced
¼ cup nonfat dry milk powder
3 tablespoons superfine flour,
  such as Wondra

¼ teaspoon salt
Several dashes of white pepper
2 cups low-fat milk
1 tablespoon chopped fresh
  chives or 1 teaspoon
  freeze-dried

Cook the cauliflower in boiling salted water to which you've added white vinegar until tender-crisp, about 3 minutes. Drain.

In a large saucepan, melt the butter and sauté the shallot until it's sizzling and fragrant, 1 to 2 minutes. Whisk the dry milk, flour, salt, and pepper into the liquid milk until well blended. Pour the milk into the saucepan and cook over medium heat, stirring constantly, until the sauce bubbles and thickens, about 5 minutes. Stir in the chives and cauliflower. Continue to simmer over very low heat for 3 minutes, stirring often.

Kilocalories 127 Kc • Protein 7 gm • Fat 4 gm • Percent of calories from fat 30% • Cholesterol 13 mg • Dietary fiber 4 gm • Sodium 234 mg • Calcium 189 mg

CREAMED CAULIFLOWER WITH PEAS: Follow the preceding recipe. Cook 2 cups shelled fresh or frozen peas in boiling salted water for 3 minutes. Drain. Stir into the cream sauce with the cauliflower.

MAKES 6 SERVINGS

Kilocalories 124 Kc • Protein 8 gm • Fat 3 gm • Percent of calories from fat 22% • Cholesterol 9 mg • Dietary fiber 5 gm • Sodium 158 mg • Calcium 138 mg

CREAMED CAULIFLOWER WITH ACORN SQUASH:

3 small acorn squash, halved and seeded
Ground nutmeg for sprinkling

Creamed Cauliflower (page 216)
6 tablespoons grated Parmesan cheese

Preheat the oven to 400 degrees F.

Put the squash into a baking dish, cut sides up, and sprinkle them with nutmeg. Pour in 1 inch of water. Bake the squash until tender, about 45 minutes.

Fill the squash halves with creamed cauliflower. Sprinkle each half with 1 tablespoon grated Parmesan cheese and return to the oven until the top is golden, 15 minutes, or, if the cauliflower was made ahead, until it's piping hot throughout, 25 to 30 minutes.

MAKES 6 SIDE-DISH SERVINGS

Kilocalories 150 Kc • Protein 9 gm • Fat 5 gm • Percent of calories from fat 26% • Cholesterol 13 mg • Dietary fiber 4 gm • Sodium 254 mg • Calcium 231 mg

Creamed Corn with Scallion Greens

■

MAKES 4 SERVINGS

One of the ultimate comfort foods, creamed corn makes a succulent side dish with meat loaf, such as Turkey Loaf with Shell Beans (pags 131).

3 cups fresh (about 6 ears) or
  frozen corn kernels
1 tablespoon unsalted butter
3 tablespoons nonfat dry milk
  powder
3 tablespoons superfine flour,
  such as Wondra

¼ teaspoon salt
Several dashes of white pepper
1½ cups low-fat milk
2 tablespoons chopped
  scallion tops

Combine the corn, ½ cup water, and butter in a saucepan. Bring to a simmer, cover, and cook until the corn is tender, about 5 minutes. Do not drain.

Blend the dry milk, flour, salt, and white pepper into the liquid milk. Pour all at once into the corn and cook over medium-high heat, stirring constantly, until the sauce bubbles and thickens, about 5 minutes. Simmer over very low heat for 3 minutes, stirring often. Stir in the scallion greens.

Kilocalories 195 Kc • Protein 7 gm • Fat 5 gm • Percent of calories from fat 23% • Cholesterol 15 mg • Dietary fiber 3 gm • Sodium 205 mg • Calcium 135 mg

CREAMED CORN WITH TOMATOES AND HERBS: Follow the preceding recipe, adding 1 ripe seeded diced tomato to the saucepan with the corn. Substitute 1 tablespoon chopped fresh marjoram and 1 teaspoon chopped fresh thyme for the scallions.

Kilocalories 201 Kc • Protein 8 gm • Fat 6 gm • Percent of calories from fat 23% • Cholesterol 15 mg • Dietary fiber 3 gm • Sodium 207 mg • Calcium 140 mg

Corn with Barley and Bell Pepper

Besides being a good source of antioxidant zinc, barley's soluble fiber makes it as heart-healthy a grain food as oats.

3 cups vegetable or chicken
   stock (pages 11, 10) or canned
   low-sodium broth
½ cup pearl barley
1 tablespoon olive oil
1 red bell pepper, diced
4 scallions, chopped

2 cups fresh or frozen corn
   kernels
½ teaspoon ground cumin
¼ teaspoon salt
⅛ teaspoon cayenne
1 tablespoon minced fresh
   cilantro

In a saucepan, heat the stock to boiling, add the barley, and simmer until it's tender, about 30 minutes. Meanwhile, heat the oil in a large skillet, and sauté the bell pepper and scallions until sizzling and fragrant, about 3 minutes. Add the corn, cumin, salt, cayenne, and ½ cup of the barley broth. Cover and simmer 5 minutes. Drain the barley and add it to the corn. Stir in the cilantro. Let stand 5 minutes to combine the flavors before serving.

Kilocalories 237 Kc • Protein 6 gm • Fat 5 gm • Percent of calories from fat 17% • Cholesterol 0 mg • Dietary fiber 6 gm • Sodium 185 mg • Calcium 20 mg

CORN WITH BARLEY AND BLACK BEANS: Follow the preceding recipe. Stir in 1 cup homemade (page 16) or canned low-sodium black beans with the barley and heat through.

Kilocalories 299 Kc • Protein 10 gm • Fat 5 gm • Percent of calories from fat 14% • Cholesterol 0 mg • Dietary fiber 9 gm • Sodium 186 mg • Calcium 43 mg

Kale with Mushrooms

Recent research has shown kale to be one of the most potent antioxidant foods.

2 tablespoons olive oil
5 ounces mushrooms, cleaned
  and sliced
1 medium yellow onion,
  chopped
1 garlic clove, finely chopped
1 large bunch kale, washed,
  trimmed, and coarsely
  chopped (about 1 pound)

1 cup vegetable or chicken stock
  (pages 11, 10) or canned low-
  sodium broth
⅛ teaspoon salt
Freshly ground black pepper

Heat the oil in a 12-inch skillet and fry the mushrooms over medium-high heat until their liquid evaporates and they begin to brown, about 5 minutes. Lower the heat, add the onion and garlic, and continue to cook until the onion begins to soften, 3 minutes. Add the kale and stock. Bring to a simmer and cook, covered, until the kale is tender, 8 to 10 minutes. Season with the salt and pepper to taste.

Kilocalories 140 Kc • Protein 5 gm • Fat 8 gm • Percent of calories from fat 48% • Cholesterol 0 mg • Dietary fiber 4 gm • Sodium 118 mg • Calcium 112 mg

ANTIOXIDANT POWER

Colcannon with Kale and Leeks

MAKES 6 SERVINGS

This is based on the traditional Irish dish, but made with oil instead of butter.

2 tablespoons olive oil
2 small leeks, sliced lengthwise, washed, and chopped
½ pound kale, washed, stemmed, and coarsely chopped
1½ cups vegetable or chicken stock (pages 11, 10) or canned low-sodium broth

4 large russet potatoes, peeled and cut into 1-inch chunks (1½ to 1¾ pounds)
1 tablespoon white vinegar
½ cup nonfat plain yogurt
¼ teaspoon salt
¼ teaspoon white pepper

In a large pot, heat the oil and "sweat" the leeks over very low heat for 10 minutes, or until they are soft and lightly colored. Add the kale and stock. Cover and simmer until the kale is very tender, about 10 minutes. Drain the vegetables, reserving the stock.

Boil the potatoes in salted water to cover, to which you've added the vinegar, until they are quite tender, about 8 minutes. Drain and dry the potatoes for a minute over low heat. Mash the potatoes. Whip in the yogurt, salt, and white pepper. Add enough of the reserved stock to make the mixture as creamy as you wish. Blend in the kale and leeks.

Kilocalories 184 Kc • Protein 6 gm • Fat 5 gm • Percent of calories from fat 24% • Cholesterol 0 mg • Dietary fiber 4 gm • Sodium 144 mg • Calcium 107 mg

COLCANNON WITH CABBAGE AND BROWNED ONIONS: Follow the preceding recipe, substituting 1 cup chopped onions for the leeks. Sauté them until they're nicely browned, 5 to 7 minutes, before adding the cabbage and stock. Use half a large head of cabbage, shredded, in place of the kale, and cook slightly less, until just tender, 5 to 6 minutes.

Kilocalories 172 Kc • Protein 6 gm • Fat 5 gm • Percent of calories from fat 25% • Cholesterol 0 mg • Dietary fiber 4 gm • Sodium 139 mg • Calcium 89 mg

Stewed Collards with Tomatoes

These savory greens can be spooned over hot rice or served plain in bowls. Pancetta is usually sliced in rounds, like Canadian bacon, and is sold at many supermarket deli counters.

2 tablespoons olive oil
2 (¼-inch thick) slices pancetta (Italian bacon)
1 medium yellow onion, chopped
2 cups seeded chopped ripe or drained and seeded canned tomatoes

1 tablespoon minced fresh flat-leaf parsley
Freshly ground black pepper
1 bunch collards, washed and coarsely chopped (¾ pound)

In a large skillet, heat the oil and fry the pancetta until it's brown and crisp, 3 to 5 minutes. Remove the pancetta and pat it with paper towels to remove excess fat. Chop the pancetta.

Clean out and dry the skillet. Add the remaining tablespoon of oil and fry the onion until it is lightly colored, 5 minutes. Add the tomatoes, parsley, and pepper to taste. Cook, uncovered, stirring often, until slightly reduced but not dry, 5 to 10 minutes.

Add the collards and pancetta. Cover and simmer over very low heat until the collards are quite tender, about 10 to 15 minutes.

Kilocalories 128 Kc • Protein 3 gm • Fat 8 gm • Percent of calories from fat 54% • Cholesterol 3 mg • Dietary fiber 4 gm • Sodium 64 mg • Calcium 30 mg

Chard with Brown Rice, Feta, and Black Olives

These greens have a Greek influence. It's worth looking for a source of fresh feta cheese, available in some small ethnic stores—it's much less salty than the feta sold in supermarkets. Red-ribbed chard can be substituted for white-ribbed; it has a slightly stronger flavor.

1 bunch white-ribbed chard
   (¾ pound)
½ cup chicken stock (page 10)
   or canned low-sodium broth
1 cup cooked brown rice (follow
   the package directions)

½ cup crumbled fresh feta
   cheese
½ cup pitted kalamata olives

Wash the chard well and cut the leaves roughly into 2-inch pieces. If the stems are large, cut them into 1-inch pieces. Put the chard in a large pot with the broth and bring to a boil. Lower the heat and simmer, covered, until tender, 10 to 15 minutes. Stir in the rice, cheese, and olives, and keep the mixture warm for 2 to 3 minutes before serving.

Kilocalories 165 Kc • Protein 6 gm • Fat 9 gm • Percent of calories from fat 50% • Cholesterol 28 mg • Dietary fiber 1 gm • Sodium 595 mg • Calcium 165 mg

VEGETABLE AND FRUIT SIDE DISHES

"Shuffled" Escarole with Cannellini

Greens cooked with oil, garlic, and very little liquid need to be stirred frequently . . . therefore "shuffled."

2 tablespoons olive oil
2 garlic cloves, finely chopped
1 bunch escarole, washed
  and cut into thirds (about
  ¾ pound)
1 cup peeled seeded chopped
  fresh tomatoes
2 cups homemade cannellini
  (white kidney beans) (page 16)
  or canned low-sodium
  cannellini, drained and rinsed

1 tablespoon minced fresh basil
  or 1 teaspoon dried
Salt and freshly ground black
  pepper

Heat the oil in a 12-inch skillet and sauté the garlic until it sizzles, about 1 minute. Immediately add the escarole and ½ cup water, cover, and simmer until the vegetable is wilted, 3 to 5 minutes. Add the tomatoes, beans, and basil, and simmer, uncovered, stirring often, for 5 to 8 minutes, until the escarole is tender. Season with salt and pepper to taste.

Kilocalories 208 Kc • Protein 10 gm • Fat 7 gm • Percent of calories from fat 31% • Cholesterol 0 mg • Dietary fiber 9 gm • Sodium 28 mg • Calcium 81 mg

ANTIOXIDANT POWER

Mushrooms and Peppers with Rosemary

MAKES 4 SERVINGS

This quick sauté goes very well with braised chicken breasts or seared tuna.

2 tablespoons olive oil
10 ounces button mushrooms, cleaned, whole, stems trimmed
1 large red bell pepper, seeded and cut into 1-inch chunks
1 large green bell pepper, seeded and cut into 1-inch chunks

2 large shallots, sliced
2 teaspoons chopped fresh rosemary or ½ teaspoon dried
Salt and freshly ground black pepper

Heat the oil in a 12-inch nonstick skillet and stir-fry the mushrooms until the caps begin to brown, 5 minutes. Add the peppers and shallots. Continue to fry over medium heat, stirring often, until the peppers are tender-crisp, 3 to 4 minutes. Stir in the rosemary during the last minute. Season the dish with salt and pepper to taste.

Kilocalories 88 Kc • Protein 2 gm • Fat 7 gm • Percent of calories from fat 67% • Cholesterol 0 mg • Dietary fiber 2 gm • Sodium 4 mg • Calcium 10 mg

VEGETABLE AND FRUIT SIDE DISHES

225

Peas, Mushrooms, and Radicchio

The slightly bitter taste of radicchio and the sweetness of peas are a flavorful contrast in this colorful side dish.

2 tablespoons olive oil
¼ cup chopped shallots
5 ounces small white
   mushrooms, cleaned, trimmed,
   and sliced
2 cups shredded radicchio
   (½ head)

2 cups shelled fresh or
   frozen peas
½ cup chicken stock (page 10)
   or canned low-sodium broth
Salt and freshly ground black
   pepper

Heat the oil in a 10-inch skillet and sauté the shallots until they begin to soften, 3 minutes. Add the mushrooms and radicchio and stir-fry over medium-high heat until the mushrooms begin to brown, 5 minutes. Add the peas and stock. Cover and simmer until the peas are tender, 5 minutes. Season with salt and pepper to taste.

Kilocalories 124 Kc • Protein 4 gm • Fat 7 gm • Percent of calories from fat 49% • Cholesterol 0 mg • Dietary fiber 4 gm • Sodium 161 mg • Calcium 6 mg

Braised Peas, Red Bell Pepper, and Shallots

Fresh mint is so far superior to dried that it's worthwhile to keep a pot of the herb growing on a sunny windowsill. It's a hardy plant that needs little encouragement to flourish.

1 tablespoon olive oil
2 shallots, chopped
1 small red bell pepper, seeded and diced
3 cups shelled fresh or frozen peas [1 (1-pound) bag]

1 teaspoon chopped fresh mint or ¼ teaspoon dried
½ teaspoon chopped fresh thyme or a pinch dried
Salt and freshly ground black pepper

Heat the oil in a medium skillet, and sauté the shallots and bell pepper until the vegetables are tender, about 5 minutes. Add the peas, cover, and braise over low heat until the peas are tender, 5 to 7 minutes, stirring often. (The other vegetables should supply sufficient moisture.) Stir in the fresh mint and thyme. (If using dried herbs, add them earlier during the braising.) Season with salt and pepper to taste.

Kilocalories 124 Kc • Protein 6 gm • Fat 4 gm • Percent of calories from fat 27% • Cholesterol 0 mg • Dietary fiber 6 gm • Sodium 6 mg • Calcium 33 mg

VEGETABLE AND FRUIT SIDE DISHES

Snow Peas with Sesame

You'll find snow peas with other Asian produce, such as fresh bean sprouts, in many supermarkets.

2 teaspoons sesame seeds
1 teaspoon vegetable oil
4 scallions, sliced diagonally
  into 1-inch pieces

¾ pound fresh snow peas, stem
  ends trimmed, or 1 (10-ounce)
  package frozen snow peas
1 teaspoon sesame oil

In a dry medium saucepan, toast the sesame seeds over very low heat until they just begin to turn golden, about 1 minute. Immediately remove them from the heat and transfer to a small bowl.

In the same saucepan, heat the oil and sauté the scallions for 2 minutes. Add the snow peas and ¼ cup water, cover, and simmer until they are tender-crisp, 3 to 5 minutes. (If you are using frozen snow peas, you will have to sacrifice the crispness and settle for tender.) Transfer to a serving dish and toss with the sesame oil. Sprinkle the sesame seeds on top.

Kilocalories 64 Kc • Protein 2 gm • Fat 3 gm • Percent of calories from fat 39% • Cholesterol 0 mg • Dietary fiber 3 gm • Sodium 9 mg • Calcium 51 mg

Bell Pepper Medley with Fresh Herbs

MAKES 4 SERVINGS

This quick dish is chock-full of vitamin C. It makes a pleasing accompaniment to a lunch omelet. And leftovers make a great sandwich.

2 tablespoons olive oil
1 large onion, separated
  into rings
1 red bell pepper, seeded and
  cut into strips
1 yellow bell pepper, seeded and
  cut into strips
1 green bell pepper, seeded and
  cut into strips

2 tablespoons red wine vinegar
¼ teaspoon salt
⅛ teaspoon freshly ground black
  pepper
1 teaspoon chopped fresh
  tarragon
1 teaspoon chopped fresh thyme
1 teaspoon chopped fresh
  parsley

Heat the oil in a large skillet, and sauté the onion and peppers until they are tender and lightly colored, 7 to 10 minutes. Toss with the remaining ingredients.

Kilocalories 90 Kc • Protein 1 gm • Fat 7 gm • Percent of calories from fat 66% • Cholesterol 0 mg • Dietary fiber 2 gm • Sodium 148 mg • Calcium 15 mg

Fruit 'n Nut Stuffed Sweet Potatoes

MAKES **8** SERVINGS

Here's some make-ahead magic with a sweet appeal to kids of all ages.

4 large sweet potatoes
¼ cup chopped unsalted pecans
2 tablespoons dried sweetened
  cranberries

2 tablespoons dark brown sugar
2 tablespoons unsalted butter,
  melted
8 pecan halves

Preheat the oven to 400 degrees F.

Pierce the potatoes in several places with a fork and place them in a baking dish. Bake until tender, 45 minutes to 1 hour. Let them cool until they can be handled.

Cut the potatoes in half lengthwise and scoop out the flesh into a bowl. Leave about ¼ inch of potato in the shells to strengthen them, and reserve the shells. Mash the potatoes and blend in the chopped nuts, cranberries, sugar, and butter. Stuff the shells with the mixture and garnish each with a pecan half. Put them into a baking pan. If made ahead, refrigerate until ready to cook.

Preheat the oven to 350 degrees F. Bake until piping hot, about 20 minutes—30 to 35 minutes if they have been refrigerated.

Kilocalories 138 Kc • Protein 1 gm • Fat 7 gm • Percent of calories from fat 41% • Cholesterol 8 mg • Dietary fiber 2 gm • Sodium 8 mg • Calcium 22 mg

Sweet Potatoes with Red Bell Peppers

MAKES 4 SERVINGS

3 large sweet potatoes, peeled
and cut into 1-inch chunks
2 tablespoons olive oil
3 red bell peppers, seeded and
cut into 1-inch chunks
1 large yellow onion, chopped

1 teaspoon chopped fresh sage
or $\frac{1}{4}$ teaspoon dried sage
leaves (not ground)
$\frac{1}{4}$ teaspoon salt
$\frac{1}{8}$ teaspoon freshly ground black
pepper

Steam the potatoes until tender, about 12 minutes.

In a large skillet, heat the oil and sauté the bell peppers and onion, stirring often, until tender, 5 to 7 minutes. Add the potatoes and heat through. Season with the sage, salt, and pepper.

Kilocalories 178 Kc • Protein 2 gm • Fat 7 gm • Percent of calories from fat 34% • Cholesterol 0 mg • Dietary fiber 4 gm • Sodium 156 mg • Calcium 40 mg

VEGETABLE AND FRUIT SIDE DISHES

Sweet Potatoes, Peppers, and Prosciutto

■

MAKES 4 SERVINGS

This is the perfect side dish to serve with a roasted loin of veal.

3 large sweet potatoes, peeled
  and cut into 1-inch chunks
2 tablespoons olive oil
3 Italian frying peppers, seeded
  and cut into 1-inch chunks
1 garlic clove, finely chopped

½ teaspoon chopped fresh
  rosemary or a pinch of dried
¼ teaspoon freshly ground black
  pepper
6 to 8 thin slices prosciutto,
  shredded (⅛ pound)

Steam the potatoes until tender, about 12 minutes.

In a large skillet, heat the oil and sauté the peppers until tender, about 5 minutes. Add the garlic during the last minute. Add the potatoes and heat through. Season with the rosemary and pepper. Gently toss with the prosciutto.

Kilocalories 172 Kc • Protein 4 gm • Fat 7 gm • Percent of calories from fat 38% • Cholesterol 7 mg • Dietary fiber 3 gm • Sodium 126 mg • Calcium 30 mg

Sweet Potato Casserole

■

Here's an easy casserole to cook alongside a roast chicken or turkey.

3 pounds sweet potatoes, peeled
  and sliced into ¼-inch-thick
  rounds (5 to 6)
2 tablespoons olive oil
1 large yellow onion, chopped
1 green bell pepper, seeded
  and diced
3 tablespoons unbleached all-
  purpose flour
½ cup nonfat dry milk powder

1 teaspoon chopped fresh thyme
  or ¼ teaspoon dried
¼ teaspoon salt
⅛ teaspoon freshly ground black
  pepper
2 cups vegetable or chicken
  stock (pages 11, 10) or canned
  low-sodium broth
½ cup seasoned bread crumbs

Parboil the potatoes in boiling salted water to cover for 3 minutes. Drain and transfer them to a 2-quart gratin dish or casserole.

In a medium saucepan, heat the oil and sauté the onion and bell pepper until they are lightly colored, 3 to 5 minutes. Stir in the flour and cook over low heat for 3 minutes; it should not brown. Whisk the dry milk, thyme, and seasonings into the stock and heat it to scalding in a separate pan. Pour the hot broth into the onion–green pepper roux and stir constantly over medium-high heat until the mixture bubbles, 2 to 3 minutes. Reduce the heat and simmer for 1 minute. Pour the sauce over the potatoes. Sprinkle with the crumbs.

Bake in the middle of the oven until the potatoes are very tender, 30 to 40 minutes.

Kilocalories 326 Kc • Protein 6 gm • Fat 5 gm • Percent of calories from fat 14% • Cholesterol 0 mg • Dietary fiber 8 gm • Sodium 160 mg • Calcium 100 mg

SWEET POTATO AND PARSNIP CASSEROLE: Follow the preceding recipe, substituting sliced parsnips for half of the sweet potatoes.

Kilocalories 306 Kc • Protein 6 gm • Fat 5 gm • Percent of calories from fat 15% • Cholesterol 0 mg • Dietary fiber 9 gm • Sodium 160 mg • Calcium 112 mg

VEGETABLE AND FRUIT SIDE DISHES

233

Sweet Potatoes with Fennel and Garlic

Fennel gives sweet potatoes a deliciously different flavor.

2 tablespoons olive oil
1 fennel bulb, cored and cut into ½-inch-thick slices
2 garlic cloves, chopped
1 (1-pound) can Italian plum tomatoes with juice

2 pounds sweet potatoes, peeled and cut into 2-inch chunks (3 to 4)
¼ teaspoon salt
Freshly ground black pepper

Preheat the oven to 400 degrees F.

Heat the oil in a Dutch oven or any range-to-oven pan and sauté the fennel until it's lightly colored, 5 minutes. Add the garlic and cook 1 minute longer. Add the tomatoes, sweet potatoes, salt, and pepper to taste.

Bring to a boil, cover, and transfer to the oven. Bake for 20 minutes. Uncover and bake until the vegetables are tender, about 5 more minutes.

Kilocalories 334 Kc • Protein 5 gm • Fat 7 gm • Percent of calories from fat 19% • Cholesterol 0 mg • Dietary fiber 9 gm • Sodium 193 mg • Calcium 114 mg

Spiced, Mashed Sweet Potatoes

MAKES 6 SERVINGS

When baking sweet potatoes, place them on a baking dish or pie pan to save the oven from sugary burns.

3 pounds sweet potatoes (5 to 6)
2 tablespoons unsalted butter, cut into pieces
1 cup nonfat plain yogurt
½ teaspoon ground cardamom

¼ teaspoon ground allspice
¼ teaspoon ground nutmeg
¼ teaspoon salt
¼ teaspoon white pepper

Preheat the oven to 400 degrees F. Pierce the potatoes with a fork in several places, and bake until very tender, 45 minutes to 1 hour.

When they can be handled, peel and mash the potatoes. Whisk in the remaining ingredients and beat until fluffy. A handheld electric mixer makes this task easier. Transfer the potatoes to a buttered 2-quart casserole.

When ready to finish, preheat the oven to 350 degrees F. Bake the casserole until the potatoes are heated through and lightly colored on top, about 20 minutes (35 minutes if the dish has been refrigerated).

Kilocalories 273 Kc • Protein 6 gm • Fat 2 gm • Percent of calories from fat 7% • Cholesterol 5 mg • Dietary fiber 7 gm • Sodium 150 mg • Calcium 140 mg

VEGETABLE AND FRUIT SIDE DISHES

Gratin of Gold and Sweet Potatoes with Leeks

MAKES **6** SERVINGS

Yellow potatoes, such as Yukon Gold, have a particularly mellow flavor that's ideally suited to this dish, but if you can't find them, white potatoes can be substituted.

3 medium leeks, white part only (1 bunch)
2 tablespoons olive oil
3 teaspoons unsalted butter
4 large yellow potatoes, peeled and sliced into ½-inch-thick rounds
2 large sweet potatoes, peeled and sliced into ½-inch-thick rounds

3 tablespoons unbleached all-purpose flour
¼ cup nonfat dry milk powder
¼ teaspoon salt
¼ teaspoon white pepper
2 cups low-fat milk, heated
1 cup fresh bread crumbs from 1 slice Italian bread
Paprika

Preheat the oven to 375 degrees F.

Cut the white part of the leeks in half lengthwise and wash between the layers. Spin or shake dry. In a saucepan, heat the oil with 1 teaspoon of butter and "sweat" the leeks (sauté over very low heat) until they are soft and tender, 10 minutes.

Parboil both kinds of potatoes together in boiling salted water until they are barely tender, 5 minutes. Drain well.

When the leeks are cooked, stir the flour into them and cook over very low heat, stirring often, for 3 minutes. Whisk the dry milk, salt, and pepper into the liquid milk, and heat it in a separate saucepan or in a microwave-safe pitcher in the microwave. Pour the hot milk all at once into the leeks, and stir constantly over medium-high heat until the mixture is thick and bubbling, 2 to 3 minutes. Reduce the heat to low and continue cooking for 2 minutes.

Arrange half the potatoes in an oiled 13 × 9-inch gratin pan or glass or ceramic baking dish. Pour half the leeks and sauce over the potatoes. Repeat with the remaining potatoes, leeks, and sauce. Sprinkle with the bread crumbs and dot with the remaining 2 teaspoons butter. Add a few dashes of paprika. Bake in the top third of the oven until tender, golden, and crusty, about 30 minutes.

Kilocalories 223 Kc • Protein 6 gm • Fat 8 gm • Percent of calories from fat 30% • Cholesterol 9 mg • Dietary fiber 3 gm • Sodium 190 mg • Calcium 167 mg

Sweet Potatoes and Carrots with Dried Fruits

MAKES 8 SERVINGS

A meatless version of tzimmes, *a sweet beef-and-vegetable stew often served at* Sukkoth, *the Jewish Feast of Tabernacles.*

6 large carrots, sliced into
  ½-inch pieces
6 sweet potatoes, peeled and cut
  into 1-inch chunks
12 dried apricot halves, cut in half
1 cup pitted prunes
2 tablespoons brown sugar

½ teaspoon ground ginger
¼ teaspoon salt
⅛ teaspoon freshly ground black
  pepper
1 cup or more hot vegetable
  stock (page 11) or canned low-
  sodium broth

Preheat the oven to 350 degrees F.
  Parboil the carrots in boiling salted water for 5 minutes. Drain.
  Combine the sweet potatoes, carrots, apricots, prunes, sugar, ginger, salt, pepper, and stock in a Dutch oven or heavy casserole. Bake, covered, until nearly tender, about 45 minutes. Stir once gently. Uncover and bake 15 minutes longer, until slightly crusty on top. Add more stock if the dish seems too dry.

Kilocalories 197 Kc • Protein 3 gm • Fat .40 gm • Percent of calories from fat 1% • Cholesterol 0 mg • Dietary fiber 6 gm • Sodium 36 mg • Calcium 56 mg

Sweet and White Potato Pancakes

MAKES 2 SERVINGS

Applesauce makes a traditional topping for these tasty cakes. A food processor, using the grater blade, takes the work out of grating potatoes; for pancakes, they must be grated finely enough to hold together when pressed.

1 large sweet potato, peeled and grated
1 large russet potato, peeled and grated
1 tablespoon finely minced onion

2 tablespoons unbleached all-purpose flour
¼ teaspoon salt
⅛ teaspoon white pepper
Dash of ground nutmeg
2 tablespoons vegetable oil

Drain the potatoes well, pressing out all excess moisture. Blend together the potatoes, onion, flour, salt, pepper, and nutmeg. Shape into 6 flat cakes.

Heat 1 tablespoon of oil in a 12-inch nonstick skillet, and fry the cakes until they are crisp and brown, about 5 minutes. Add the remaining tablespoon of oil and brown the second side of the cakes, about 5 minutes. Serve hot.

Kilocalories 348 Kc • Protein 6 gm • Fat 14 gm • Percent of calories from fat 36% • Cholesterol 0 mg • Dietary fiber 6 gm • Sodium 306 mg • Calcium 45 mg

Scalloped Potatoes

Here's an old favorite in a streamlined, low-fat version.

1 tablespoon olive oil

1 large yellow onion, peeled, sliced, and separated into rings

6 medium russet potatoes, peeled and cut into ¼-inch-thick rounds

1½ cups chicken or vegetable stock (pages 10, 11) or canned low-sodium broth

¼ teaspoon salt

⅛ teaspoon freshly ground black pepper

½ cup nonfat dry milk powder

3 tablespoons superfine flour, such as Wondra

1 cup low-fat milk

2 tablespoons grated Parmesan cheese

Preheat the oven to 375 degrees F.

Put the oil and onion into a medium gratin dish, and bake until the onion is sizzling and yellow, 5 to 7 minutes. Remove the dish from the oven.

Put the potatoes, stock, salt, and pepper into a large saucepan. Bring to a boil, cover, and simmer for 5 minutes. Remove the potatoes with a slotted spoon and arrange them in the gratin dish with the onions.

Whisk the dry milk and flour into the liquid milk. Add to the stock and bring to a boil, stirring constantly, until the sauce bubbles and thickens slightly, about 5 minutes. Simmer 1 to 2 minutes. Pour the sauce over the potatoes. Sprinkle with the cheese and bake for 30 to 35 minutes, until the potatoes are very tender and the top is golden.

Kilocalories 238 Kc • Protein 9 gm • Fat 4 gm • Percent of calories from fat 15% • Cholesterol 5 mg • Dietary fiber 4 gm • Sodium 176 mg • Calcium 123 mg

VEGETABLE AND FRUIT SIDE DISHES

Garlicky Scalloped Potatoes

___

MAKES **6** SERVINGS

These potatoes have even less fat than the preceding recipe, and are richly flavored with roasted garlic.

1 whole garlic bulb
6 large red potatoes, peeled and
    sliced into ¼-inch-thick
    rounds
1 scant teaspoon chopped fresh
    rosemary or ¼ teaspoon dried

About ¼ teaspoon salt in total
Freshly ground black pepper
About 1½ cups hot chicken or
    vegetable stock (pages 10, 11)
    or canned low-sodium broth

Preheat the oven to 375 degrees F.

Cut off the top of the garlic bulb and wrap it in foil. Bake for 45 minutes, or until soft when pressed. Cool the garlic enough to handle. Squeeze the garlic cloves out of their peels. Chop the garlic.

Parboil the potatoes in boiling salted water for 5 minutes. Drain.

Layer a third of the potato slices in an oiled 2-quart casserole. Sprinkle with half the garlic and rosemary. Add a little salt and pepper. Make a second layer of a third of the potatoes. Add the rest of the garlic and rosemary, plus more salt and pepper. Top with the remaining potatoes and salt and pepper. Add enough hot stock to reach almost to the top layer of potatoes. Bake until the potatoes are golden and very tender, about 30 minutes.

Kilocalories 156 Kc • Protein 6 gm • Fat .45 gm • Percent of calories from fat 3% • Cholesterol 0 mg • Dietary fiber 4 gm • Sodium 114 mg • Calcium 29 mg

Red Potatoes Gratin

MAKES 6 SERVINGS

Use a shallow gratin dish for this potato casserole with melted cheese topping.

6 large red potatoes
1 large yellow onion
1 tablespoon olive oil
2½ cups chicken or vegetable stock (pages 10, 11) or canned low-sodium broth
¼ teaspoon salt

⅛ teaspoon freshly ground black pepper
2 tablespoons unbleached all-purpose flour
¾ cup shredded Gruyère or Asiago cheese

Preheat the oven to 375 degrees F.

Scrub the potatoes, removing any sprouts, and cut them, unpeeled, into ¼-inch slices. Peel and slice the onion, separating the slices into rings.

In a large saucepan, heat the oil and sauté the onion until it's soft and yellow, 3 to 5 minutes. Add the potatoes, 2 cups of stock, the salt, and pepper. Bring to a boil, cover, and simmer until the potatoes are nearly tender, 5 minutes. With a slotted spoon, remove the potatoes and onions, and transfer them to a 2-quart gratin dish. Keep the potato stock at a simmer.

Pour the remaining ½ cup cold stock into a jar, add the flour, cover tightly, and shake until blended. Pour the flour mixture all at once into the potato stock and cook over medium-high heat, stirring constantly, until the sauce is slightly thickened and bubbling, 2 to 3 minutes. Simmer the sauce, stirring often, for 3 minutes.

Pour the sauce over the potatoes, using just enough so that the top layer is not covered. Sprinkle with cheese and bake for 30 to 35 minutes, until the potatoes are very tender and the top is golden.

Kilocalories 233 Kc • Protein 11 gm • Fat 5 gm • Percent of calories from fat 19% • Cholesterol 8 mg • Dietary fiber 4 gm • Sodium 146 mg • Calcium 173 mg

VEGETABLE AND FRUIT SIDE DISHES

Mashed Potatoes with Caramelized Onions

MAKES 4 SERVINGS

If you're cooking a roast of any kind—beef, pork, lamb, or chicken—for the same meal, simply put the onion in the pan around the meat and scoop it out with a slotted spoon when browned. This flavors both the roast and the onions deliciously. Otherwise, follow the directions below for preparing the onions.

1 large onion, peeled and sliced
   into ½-inch-thick rounds
2 teaspoons olive oil
6 to 8 russet potatoes, peeled
   and cut into 1-inch chunks
   (2 pounds)
1 teaspoon white vinegar

⅔ cup nonfat plain yogurt at
   room temperature
¼ teaspoon white pepper
¼ teaspoon salt
1 tablespoon minced fresh flat-
   leaf parsley

Preheat the oven to 350 degrees F.

Put the onion into a small casserole with the oil, turn to coat all sides, and bake until browned but not burned, about 30 minutes.

Put the potatoes in a large saucepan with water to cover. Add the vinegar. Boil the potatoes until fork-tender, about 8 minutes. Drain and put them back in the saucepan over warm heat to dry out the last of the moisture. Mash the potatoes. Whip in the yogurt, pepper, salt, and parsley. Stir in the browned onions, keep warm 3 minutes or so to blend the flavors, then serve.

Kilocalories 284 Kc • Protein 10 gm • Fat 3 gm • Percent of calories from fat 9% • Cholesterol 0 mg • Dietary fiber 6 gm • Sodium 185 mg • Calcium 114 mg

MASHED POTATOES WITH CHILI BEANS: Here's a tasty way to use leftover mashed potatoes. Preheat the oven to 350 degrees F. Using the mashed potatoes from the preceding recipe, layer 1½ to 2 cups potatoes (or whatever amount is left over) in an oiled gratin pan. Mix 1 cup homemade (page 16) or canned drained and rinsed low-sodium red kidney beans with 2 tablespoons chili sauce and spread them over the potatoes. Bake until piping hot throughout, 20 to 25 minutes.

This makes a nice meatless lunch dish for two or a brunch accompaniment to scrambled eggs for four.

Kilocalories 351 Kc • Protein 16 gm • Fat 2 gm • Percent of calories from fat 6% • Cholesterol 0 mg • Dietary fiber 10 gm • Sodium 153 mg • Calcium 119 mg

Baked Pumpkin Wedges

MAKES 6 SERVINGS

Flavorful cooking pumpkins, sometimes called "sugar pumpkins," are small in size, about two pounds.

1 (2 to 2½-pound) "sugar" pumpkin, seeds removed, cut into 6 wedges

2 tablespoons unsalted butter, melted

2 tablespoons brown sugar, sifted

Ground nutmeg for sprinkling

Preheat the oven to 375 degrees F.

Make several shallow slits in each pumpkin wedge. Place the wedges in a roasting pan, cut sides up, and drizzle the butter over the slits. Sprinkle the wedges with brown sugar and nutmeg. Pour 1 cup water into the pan. Bake until the pumpkin is tender, about 45 minutes.

Kilocalories 92 Kc • Protein 2 gm • Fat 4 gm • Percent of calories from fat 37% • Cholesterol 11 mg • Dietary fiber 1 gm • Sodium 45 mg • Calcium 37 mg

Pumpkin with Tomatoes and Garlic

This recipe puts a new spin on the Halloween pumpkin.

1 tablespoon olive oil
2 garlic cloves, minced
1 (16-ounce) can Italian plum
  tomatoes, chopped, with juice
¼ teaspoon salt
Freshly ground black pepper

1½ pounds peeled diced
  pumpkin or butternut squash
  (2 pounds unpeeled)
2 tablespoon chopped fresh
  basil, 1 teaspoon basil pesto, or
  ½ teaspoon dried basil

In a 10-inch skillet, heat the oil and sauté the garlic until it's sizzling, about 1 minute. Add the tomatoes and salt and pepper to taste, and simmer, uncovered, for 5 minutes. Add the pumpkin, cover, and continue to cook until it's tender, 8 to 10 minutes. Stir in the basil.

Kilocalories 116 Kc • Protein 3 gm • Fat 4 gm • Percent of calories from fat 32% • Cholesterol 0 mg • Dietary fiber 3 gm • Sodium 16 mg • Calcium 77 mg

Pumpkin with Cashews and Ginger

■

MAKES 4 SERVINGS

When toasting nuts or seeds, remove them from the pan the second they have reached a golden color or the heat from the pan will over-brown them.

⅓ cup unsalted cashew halves
  or pieces
1 tablespoon or more
  vegetable oil
4 scallions, chopped
1 slice fresh ginger, minced

1½ pounds peeled diced
  pumpkin or Hubbard squash
  (about 2 pounds unpeeled)
½ cup chicken or vegetable
  stock (pages 10, 11) or canned
  low-sodium broth

In a dry 10-inch skillet, toast the cashews over low heat until they just start to turn golden, about 1 minute. Immediately remove them to a small dish.

Heat the oil in the same skillet, and stir-fry the scallions and ginger for 2 minutes, or until the scallions begin to brown. Add the pumpkin and continue to stir-fry for 2 minutes. If necessary, add more oil.

Add the stock, cover, and cook until the pumpkin is tender, 8 to 10 minutes. Transfer to a serving dish and sprinkle with the cashews.

Kilocalories 144 Kc • Protein 4 gm • Fat 9 gm • Percent of calories from fat 51% • Cholesterol 0 mg • Dietary fiber 1 gm • Sodium 10 mg • Calcium 45 mg

Pumpkin with Apples and Mint

Mint gives a piquant flavor to this side dish.

About 3 cups peeled diced
  pumpkin or butternut squash
  (¾ pound)
½ cup apple juice
1 tablespoon brown sugar

¼ teaspoon ground nutmeg
1 large apple, such as Rome or
  Macoun, peeled and diced
2 teaspoons chopped fresh mint
  or ½ teaspoon dried

Combine the pumpkin, apple juice, brown sugar, and nutmeg in a medium saucepan. Simmer, covered, until the pumpkin is nearly tender, 5 to 7 minutes. Add the diced apple and continue cooking until both are tender, about 5 minutes. If using dried mint, add it 1 minute before removing from the heat. If using fresh mint, stir it in after cooking.

Kilocalories 69 Kc • Protein 1 gm • Fat 0 gm • Percent of calories from fat 3% • Cholesterol 0 mg • Dietary fiber 1 gm • Sodium 5 mg • Calcium 23 mg

Spinach with Lemon and Olives

MAKES 6 SERVINGS

Serve this easy dish of greens as a side dish or as a toping for polenta (page 12).

1½ pounds or 2 (10-ounce)
  packages fresh spinach,
  washed, tough stems removed,
  and coarsely chopped
½ cup quartered or sliced pitted
  black olives

2 tablespoons olive oil
Salt and freshly ground black
  pepper
2 tablespoons fresh lemon juice

Put the spinach into a large pot with ¼ cup water. Cook over high heat until wilted, 3 to 5 minutes. Drain the spinach. Return it to the pot; add the olives and olive oil. Season with salt and pepper to taste. Heat 2 minutes, then transfer to a serving dish and toss with the lemon juice.

Kilocalories 86 Kc • Protein 3 gm • Fat 7 gm • Percent of calories from fat 63% • Cholesterol 0 mg • Dietary fiber 3 gm • Sodium 197 mg • Calcium 113 mg

Spinach with Pancetta

■

MAKES 4 SERVINGS

1 to 2 slices pancetta (Italian bacon), finely diced (about ½ cup)

1 (10-ounce) package fresh spinach, washed and chopped

¼ cup low-sodium chicken broth

Freshly ground black pepper

In a small unoiled nonstick skillet, slowly sauté the pancetta until it's brown and crisp, 3 to 5 minutes. Remove the pancetta with a slotted spoon and drain it between paper towels. Discard the fat.

In a large pot, combine the spinach and broth, and cook over medium heat until the spinach wilts, about 5 minutes. Combine the pancetta and spinach. Season with pepper to taste.

Kilocalories 46 Kc • Protein 7 gm • Fat 1 gm • Percent of calories from fat 23% • Cholesterol 10 mg • Dietary fiber 2 gm • Sodium 291 mg • Calcium 71 mg

Spinach-stuffed Baked Potatoes

MAKES 4 SERVINGS

4 large baking potatoes
1 tablespoon olive oil
1 small yellow onion, chopped
10 ounces fresh spinach, washed, tough stems removed, finely chopped
½ cup part-skim ricotta cheese
2 tablespoons grated Romano cheese
¼ teaspoon salt
⅛ teaspoon freshly ground black pepper

Preheat the oven to 400 degrees F. Scrub the potatoes, remove any sprouts, and prick them in several places with a fork. Bake the potatoes until they are fork-tender, about 1 hour. When they are cool enough to handle, scoop out the flesh into a large bowl, leaving ¼-inch-thick shells.

Heat the oil in a large saucepan and sauté the onion until it's soft and yellow, 3 to 5 minutes. Put the spinach into the same pan with 2 tablespoons of water. Cover and cook over medium heat until the spinach is wilted, about 3 minutes. Remove the spinach-onion mixture with a slotted spoon.

Mash the potato. Mash in the spinach, ricotta, grated Romano cheese, salt, and pepper. Stuff the potato shells with the mixture and put them into a shallow baking pan. At this point you can refrigerate the potatoes for several hours. When ready to finish them, reheat the oven to 400 degrees F.

Bake the potatoes until they are hot throughout and golden on top, about 20 minutes if the ingredients are still warm, 30 minutes if made ahead and refrigerated.

Kilocalories 314 Kc • Protein 14 gm • Fat 7 gm • Percent of calories from fat 21% • Cholesterol 12 mg • Dietary fiber 8 gm • Sodium 295 mg • Calcium 212 mg

Acorn Squash Stuffed with Brown Mushrooms

Brown mushrooms have a richer, earthier flavor (more like wild mushrooms) than the white button variety.

2 (1-pound) acorn squash, halved and seeded

2 tablespoons olive oil

5 ounces small portobello or any brown mushrooms, cleaned and sliced

1 shallot, chopped

1 cup fresh bread crumbs from 1 slice Italian bread

1 tablespoon chopped fresh flat-leaf parsley

1 tablespoon chopped fresh chives

⅛ teaspoon salt

Several dashes of freshly ground black pepper

About ½ cup chicken stock (page 10) or canned low-sodium broth

Preheat the oven to 400 degrees F. Place the squash in a baking dish, cut sides up, and pour in 1 inch of water. Bake until golden and tender, 40 to 45 minutes. It's all right if the water boils out.

Heat 1 tablespoon of oil in a medium skillet, and fry the mushrooms over medium-high heat until they give up their juice and begin to brown, about 5 minutes. Add the shallot to the pan during the last 2 minutes of cooking.

Mix the bread crumbs, herbs, and seasonings with the mushrooms. Add enough stock to moisten, and stuff the squash, mounding up the stuffing. Drizzle a little of the remaining oil over each. Reduce the oven heat to 350 degrees F, and bake until the stuffing browns, about 20 minutes.

Kilocalories 182 Kc • Protein 6 gm • Fat 8 gm • Percent of calories from fat 35% • Cholesterol 0 mg • Dietary fiber 5 gm • Sodium 136 mg • Calcium 95 mg

VEGETABLE AND FRUIT SIDE DISHES

Acorn Squash, Sweet Potato, and Apple Casserole

MAKES 4 SERVINGS

For Thanksgiving or any occasion, this is an attractive make-ahead casserole.

1 large acorn squash, halved and seeded

2 sweet potatoes

2 tablespoons unsalted butter, melted

2 tablespoons brown sugar

Several dashes of ground allspice and ground cinnamon

2 red cooking apples, such as Rome or Gala, cored, unpeeled, and cut into thick rounds

Preheat the oven to 400 degrees F.

Arrange the squash halves cut sides up in a baking dish. Pierce the sweet potatoes in several places with a cooking fork and place them in a pie pan. Bake the vegetables in the middle of the oven until they are tender, 45 minutes to 1 hour. Let them cool until they can be handled.

Peel and slice the squash and potatoes. Spread half the butter in a 9 × 9-inch baking dish. Make one layer of the squash, a second later of sweet potatoes, and sprinkle them with 1 tablespoon of sugar and a few dashes of the spices.

Make a layer of overlapping apple slices on top of the vegetables. Sprinkle with the remaining 1 tablespoon of sugar and more spices. Drizzle the remaining butter over all.

Reheat the oven to 375 degrees F. Bake the casserole until the apples are tender when pierced and the squash is heated through, about 25 minutes.

Kilocalories 251 Kc • Protein 5 gm • Fat 4 gm • Percent of calories from fat 12% • Cholesterol 8 mg • Dietary fiber 7 gm • Sodium 22 mg • Calcium 112 mg

ANTIOXIDANT POWER

250

Baked Butternut Squash with Maple-Walnut Apples

MAKES **6** SERVINGS

In recipes where maple syrup is used as a sweetener, I like to boost the flavor with a little concentrated maple flavoring, found in specialty stores and some supermarkets.

1 medium butternut squash, quartered lengthwise and seeded (2 pounds)
Ground nutmeg for sprinkling
½ cup unsalted walnut halves or pieces
2 large red cooking apples, such as Rome or Macoun, cored, unpeeled, and sliced into ½-inch-thick rings

¼ cup maple syrup
2 tablespoons unsalted butter, melted
¼ teaspoon natural maple flavoring (optional, but tasty)

Preheat the oven to 375 degrees F. Put the squash into a roasting pan, cut sides up, and sprinkle it with nutmeg. Add about ½ inch of water to the pan and roast the squash until tender but still firm, about 45 minutes. Remove and cool until it can be handled. Peel and slice the squash. Layer it into a buttered baking dish from which you can serve.

In a small saucepan, cover the walnuts with water and bring them to a boil. Remove from the heat. Drain and rinse.

Layer the apple rings over the squash, overlapping as necessary. Combine the maple syrup, butter, and maple flavoring, if using. Drizzle this mixture over all. Be sure to cover all the apple surfaces with the syrup.

Reheat the oven to 375 degrees F. Bake the casserole until the apples are tender when pierced and the squash is steaming hot, about 25 minutes. Baste the apples with the juices at the bottom of the casserole once during the cooking time.

Kilocalories 192 Kc • Protein 5 gm • Fat 8 gm • Percent of calories from fat 36% • Cholesterol 5 mg • Dietary fiber 4 gm • Sodium 9 mg • Calcium 68 mg

VEGETABLE AND FRUIT SIDE DISHES

251

Roasted Butternut Squash with Garlic

MAKES 4 SERVINGS

Garlic simply placed in the hollow of the squash will give quite a lot of flavor, but if you enjoy a stronger flavor, squeeze the garlic pulp over the vegetable before serving.

Salt and freshly ground black pepper
1 (2-pound) butternut squash, quartered lengthwise and seeded

4 garlic cloves, skins loosened at one end
4 teaspoons extra-virgin olive oil

Preheat the oven to 375 degrees F.

Salt and pepper the squash to taste. Arrange the squash in a baking dish, cut sides up, and pour ½ inch of water into the pan. Put a garlic clove in each squash hollow. Drizzle the oil over all.

Bake until the squash is tender, about 45 minutes.

Kilocalories 128 Kc • Protein 3 gm • Fat 5 gm • Percent of calories from fat 31% • Cholesterol 0 mg • Dietary fiber 3 gm • Sodium 10 mg • Calcium 76 mg

Sweet-and-Sour Butternut Squash

MAKES 4 SERVINGS

It's not just for juleps—fresh mint, popular in many Mediterranean countries, is a great herb to enhance sweet or bland vegetables.

½ large butternut squash,
  peeled, seeded, and cut into
  1-inch pieces (¾ to 1 pound)
2 tablespoons olive oil
2 shallots, minced
2 teaspoons sugar

¼ teaspoon salt
Freshly ground black pepper
1 tablespoon white wine vinegar
1 tablespoon chopped
  fresh mint leaves or
  ½ teaspoon dried

Steam the butternut squash until it's nearly tender but not mushy, about 12 minutes.

Heat the olive oil and sauté the shallots until they are sizzling, 1 to 2 minutes. Add the squash and continue to sauté until the vegetable is quite tender, 3 minutes. Sprinkle with sugar, salt, and pepper to taste. Season with vinegar and mint. Heat on a very low setting for 5 minutes to blend the flavors.

Kilocalories 101 Kc • Protein 1 gm • Fat 7 gm • Percent of calories from fat 58% • Cholesterol 0 mg • Dietary fiber 1 gm • Sodium 149 mg • Calcium 30 mg

VEGETABLE AND FRUIT SIDE DISHES

253

Sautéed Herbed Cherry Tomatoes

MAKES 4 SERVINGS

Fresh herbs are a "must" in this five-minute side dish.

1 tablespoon olive oil	1 teaspoon minced fresh
1 shallot, chopped	marjoram (optional)
1 pint cherry tomatoes, halved	1 teaspoon chopped fresh chives
1 teaspoon minced fresh basil	Salt and freshly ground pepper

Heat the oil in a large skillet and sauté the shallot until sizzling, 1 to 2 minutes. Add the tomatoes and stir-fry until they are slightly softened, 3 to 5 minutes. Add the herbs during the last minute. Season with salt and pepper to taste.

Kilocalories 59 Kc • Protein 1 gm • Fat 4 gm • Percent of calories from fat 53% • Cholesterol 0 mg • Dietary fiber 2 gm • Sodium 12 mg • Calcium 7 mg

Old-fashioned Stewed Tomatoes

MAKES 4 SERVINGS

Serve on the side in sauce dishes or as a topping for cooked rice.

1 tablespoon olive oil	1 teaspoon sugar
1 tablespoon unsalted butter	¼ teaspoon salt
1 small yellow onion, finely	1 tablespoon minced fresh
chopped	cilantro or 1 teaspoon dried
1 celery stalk, sliced thin	
2 pounds ripe tomatoes, peeled,	
seeded, and cut into 1-inch	
chunks, or 1 (28-ounce) can	
tomatoes with juice, chopped	

In a large skillet, heat the oil and butter and sauté the onion and celery very slowly for 5 minutes; do not brown. Add the tomatoes, sugar, and salt. Cook, uncovered, over very low heat until tender and slightly thickened, about 20 minutes. Stir in the cilantro.

Kilocalories 81 Kc • Protein 2 gm • Fat 5 gm • Percent of calories from fat 49% • Cholesterol 5 mg • Dietary fiber 2 gm • Sodium 138 mg • Calcium 16 mg

STEWED TOMATOES WITH CORN: Follow the preceding recipe, but omit the sugar and add 1½ cups fresh or frozen corn kernels and ½ teaspoon ground cumin during the last 10 minutes of cooking.

MAKES 6 SERVINGS

Kilocalories 120 Kc • Protein 3 gm • Fat 5 gm • Percent of calories from fat 35% • Cholesterol 5 mg • Dietary fiber 3 gm • Sodium 140 mg • Calcium 19 mg

STEWED TOMATOES WITH PEAS: Follow the basic stewed tomato recipe, but omit the sugar and add 1½ cups shelled fresh or frozen peas during the last 7 minutes of cooking. Substitute 2 teaspoons chopped fresh basil or ½ teaspoon dried and 1 teaspoon chopped fresh mint or ¼ teaspoon dried for the cilantro.

MAKES 6 SERVINGS

Kilocalories 108 Kc • Protein 4 gm • Fat 5 gm • Percent of calories from fat 39% • Cholesterol 5 mg • Dietary fiber 4 gm • Sodium 139 mg • Calcium 25 mg

STEWED TOMATOES WITH PEPPERS: Follow the basic stewed tomato recipe. Sauté 2 seeded diced green bell peppers and 1 seeded minced jalapeño pepper (wear rubber gloves) with the onion and celery. Omit the sugar.

MAKES 6 SERVINGS

Kilocalories 86 Kc • Protein 2 gm • Fat 5 gm • Percent of calories from fat 46% • Cholesterol 5 mg • Dietary fiber 3 gm • Sodium 138 mg • Calcium 18 mg

Sautéed Zucchini and Red Cabbage

MAKES 4 SERVINGS

Besides its great antioxidant power, cabbage offers a bonus of anti-cancer phytochemicals.

2 tablespoons olive oil

1 medium zucchini, cut into
 1-inch chunks

2 scallions, cut diagonally into
 1-inch pieces

2 cups shredded red cabbage

1 tablespoon chopped fresh flat-
 leaf parsley

¼ teaspoon salt

Freshly ground black pepper

Heat the oil in a 10-inch skillet. Sauté the zucchini, scallions, and cabbage until the vegetables are tender and the zucchini is lightly browned, 5 to 7 minutes. Season with parsley, salt, and pepper to taste.

Kilocalories 75 Kc • Protein 1 gm • Fat 7 gm • Percent of calories from fat 78% • Cholesterol 0 mg • Dietary fiber 1 gm • Sodium 151 mg • Calcium 26 mg

Stir-fried Zucchini and Bell Peppers with Rosemary Rice

MAKES 4 SERVINGS

The edible skin of the zucchini can hold a fine grit of soil, so it needs a good scrub with a vegetable brush rather than just a rinse.

1 red bell pepper, seeded and cut into triangles
1 green bell pepper, seeded and cut into triangles
2 tablespoons olive oil
¼ cup chopped shallots
1 medium zucchini, diced

2 cups cooked brown rice or white rice (use package directions)
½ teaspoon chopped fresh rosemary or ¼ teaspoon dried
Salt and freshly ground black pepper

Seed the peppers and cut them roughly into triangles. Heat the oil in a large skillet and sauté the peppers, shallots, and zucchini until they are tender-crisp, 4 to 5 minutes. Add the rice and rosemary, and salt and pepper to taste. Stir-fry another 3 minutes.

Kilocalories 189 Kc • Protein 3 gm • Fat 8 gm • Percent of calories from fat 36% • Cholesterol 0 mg • Dietary fiber 3 gm • Sodium 4 mg • Calcium 24 mg

VEGETABLE AND FRUIT SIDE DISHES

Gingered Vegetable Stir-fry

Here's a five-minute side dish for an after-work supper. Baked fish and hot rice would round out the menu.

1 tablespoon vegetable oil
2 carrots, very thinly sliced
2 celery stalks, thinly sliced
1 red bell pepper, thinly sliced
1 medium zucchini, thinly sliced
4 scallions, chopped

1 slice fresh ginger, minced
  (about 1 tablespoon)
1 tablespoon naturally brewed
  reduced-sodium soy sauce
1 teaspoon sesame oil

In a large wok or skillet, heat the vegetable oil until quite hot. Stir-fry the carrots, celery, bell pepper, zucchini, scallions, and ginger until the vegetables are tender-crisp, 3 to 5 minutes. Transfer the vegetables to a serving dish, and toss them with the soy sauce and sesame oil.

Kilocalories 78 Kc • Protein 2 gm • Fat 5 gm • Percent of calories from fat 51% • Cholesterol 0 mg • Dietary fiber 3 gm • Sodium 185 mg • Calcium 36 mg

Winter Vegetables with Butter and Mint

Fresh herbs are generally available all year in today's supermarkets. They'll keep about a week, stored and refrigerated like any leafy green vegetable (page 183).

4 medium beets
8 small boiling onions
4 small turnips, peeled and cut
  in half
8 baby carrots
1 cup vegetable or chicken stock
  (pages 11, 10) or canned low-
  sodium broth

1 tablespoon unsalted butter
Salt and white pepper
1 tablespoon chopped fresh
  mint or ½ teaspoon dried

In separate saucepans, cook the beets and onions, unpeeled, in boiling salted water until tender, about 20 minutes. Drain and cool until they can be handled. Peel the beets and cut them in half. Cut the root ends off the onions and slip them out of their skins.

In another saucepan, simmer the turnips and carrots in the stock until they are tender, about 15 minutes. Stir in the beets, onions, and butter. Season with salt and pepper to taste. Transfer the mixed vegetables to a serving dish and sprinkle with the mint before serving.

Kilocalories 168 Kc • Protein 5 gm • Fat 2 gm • Percent of calories from fat 11% • Cholesterol 4 mg • Dietary fiber 10 gm • Sodium 236 mg • Calcium 72 mg

VEGETABLE AND FRUIT SIDE DISHES

259

Mediterranean Vegetables Glazed with Balsamic Vinegar

MAKES 4 SERVINGS

Here's a simple and colorful side dish that could accompany a chicken entrée, such as Oven-Fried Chicken Breasts with Potatoes and Carrots (page 124).

2 tablespoons olive oil
1 red onion, peeled, sliced, and separated into rings
1 medium zucchini, cut into half rounds
1 large red bell pepper, seeded and cut into strips
1 large green bell pepper, seeded and cut into strips

1 large yellow bell pepper, seeded and cut into strips
2 tablespoons balsamic vinegar
Salt and freshly ground black pepper
1 tablespoon minced fresh flat-leaf parsley

Heat the oil in a 12-inch nonstick skillet and sauté the onion until it sizzles, 1 to 2 minutes. Add the zucchini and stir-fry until it begins to soften, 3 minutes. Add the peppers and continue to stir-fry until they are tender, about 5 minutes. Add the vinegar and cook, stirring, until it's reduced to a glaze, 1 to 2 minutes. Season the vegetables with salt and pepper to taste, and sprinkle with parsley.

Kilocalories 105 Kc • Protein 1 gm • Fat 7 gm • Percent of calories from fat 58% • Cholesterol 0 mg • Dietary fiber 2 gm • Sodium 5 mg • Calcium 20 mg

ANTIOXIDANT POWER

260

Ratatouille with Portobellos

Leftover ratatouille makes a superb filling for pita pockets.

Salt

1 large eggplant (about 1 pound)

3 tablespoons olive oil, or more if needed

1 red bell pepper, seeded and cut into strips

1 green bell pepper, seeded and cut into strips

3 large portobello mushroom caps, cleaned and sliced

1 large yellow onion, chopped

3 garlic cloves, chopped

2 cups fresh seeded or canned drained chopped tomatoes

1 tablespoon chopped fresh basil or 1 teaspoon dried

¼ teaspoon freshly ground black pepper

2 medium zucchini, cut into ½-inch slices, then cut into quarters (about 1 pound)

2 tablespoons chopped fresh flat-leaf parsley

Peel, slice, and salt the eggplant. Allow the slices to drain in a colander for a half hour. Rinse the slices and press them dry between paper towels. Cut the slices into quarters.

In a 12-inch nonstick skillet, heat 2 tablespoons of the oil and slowly sauté the bell peppers, mushrooms, and onion for 5 minutes. Add the remaining tablespoon of oil and the eggplant; stir-fry for 2 minutes over medium-high heat. Lower the heat, add the garlic, and sauté 1 minute longer.

Add the tomatoes, basil, ¼ teaspoon salt, and pepper, and simmer, uncovered, for 5 minutes. Add the zucchini. If the mixture seems dry, add ¼ cup of water. Cover and cook over very low heat for 15 to 20 minutes. The vegetables should be very tender but still hold their shape. Stir occasionally and gently.

Sprinkle the dish with parsley. Serve warm or at room temperature.

Kilocalories 128 Kc • Protein 3 gm • Fat 7 gm • Percent of calories from fat 47% • Cholesterol 0 mg • Dietary fiber 5 gm • Sodium 110 mg • Calcium 34 mg

VEGETABLE AND FRUIT SIDE DISHES

Whole Cranberry and Apricot Sauce

MAKES ABOUT 3 CUPS, 6 SERVINGS

This cranberry sauce has quite a different and pleasing flavor, a nice companion to any poultry dish.

1 (12- to 13-ounce) bag fresh
   cranberries, picked over and
   rinsed
½ pound chopped dried apricots

1½ cups orange juice
1 cup sugar
½ teaspoon grated orange zest

Combine all the ingredients in a large heavy saucepan. Bring to a boil, stirring to dissolve the sugar. Simmer over low heat, uncovered, stirring often, until the berries have popped and the sauce is thick, 15 to 20 minutes. When the sauce has cooled a bit, transfer it to a bowl. When cool, refrigerate. The sauce will thicken more as it cools.

Kilocalories 275 Kc • Protein 2 gm • Fat 0 gm • Percent of calories from fat 1% • Cholesterol 0 mg • Dietary fiber 6 gm • Sodium 5 mg • Calcium 28 mg

Savory Peach Side Dish

MAKES 6 SERVINGS

These sliced peaches are a nice accompaniment to a meat entrée, such as braised chicken. Fresh herbs work best in this recipe.

3 ripe peaches, peeled and
   sliced
¼ cup dry vermouth or dry
   white wine

½ teaspoon minced fresh
   rosemary
½ teaspoon minced fresh thyme
Freshly ground black pepper

Combine all the ingredients with black pepper to taste. Allow the peaches to marinate at room temperature for a half hour before serving.

Kilocalories 29 Kc • Protein 0 gm • Fat .25 gm • Percent of calories from fat 1% • Cholesterol 0 mg • Dietary fiber 1 gm • Sodium 0 mg • Calcium 5 mg

Rosy Red Applesauce

■

MAKES 1 QUART, 6 SERVINGS

This unusual applesauce makes a pleasing side dish with grilled pork chops.

1 medium beet, peeled and
   thinly sliced
4 large apples, such as Rome or
   Cortland (1¾ to 2 pounds),
   peeled, seeded, and sliced

½ cup sugar
1 tablespoon cider vinegar
1 cinnamon stick

Put the beet into a medium saucepan with 1 cup of water and simmer, covered, for 10 minutes. Add the apples, sugar, vinegar, and cinnamon stick, stirring to dissolve the sugar in the hot beet juice. Simmer, this time with the cover ajar, stirring frequently, until the apples are very tender, about 10 minutes. As the syrup cooks down, there will be a tendency to boil over, so keep the simmer very low.

Cool slightly. Remove the cinnamon stick. Puree the apples, beet, and syrup in a food processor. Chill until ready to serve.

Kilocalories 155 Kc • Protein 1 gm • Fat .47 gm • Percent of calories from fat 2% • Cholesterol 0 mg • Dietary fiber 4 gm • Sodium 24 mg • Calcium 16 mg

Breads and Muffins

The delectable aroma of baking bread just naturally draws hungry people to the table. It might be a quick bread that you can whip up in a half hour or so. Or it could be a yeast bread rising in a warm place, later to be baked to a beautiful golden brown. Or it might be a dozen tasty muffins. Whichever you choose to prepare, the special fragrance of bread in the oven evokes a part of what we mean by "memories of home."

It's heartwarming to know that those good homemade baked goods can be infused with antioxidant power as well as better-than-store-bought flavor. Choosing whole grains enriches them with vitamin E, and "fold-ins" like fresh raspberries, grated carrots, or dried apricots add vitamin C and beta-carotene as well.

Fortunately for those who indulge in an occasional baking binge, homemade breads, muffins, and coffee cakes can be frozen for two to three months and will still taste delightfully fresh when thawed. Just be sure to cool them completely and wrap them thoroughly before freezing. Unwrap before thawing.

Store-bought muffins are often so greatly sugared that they should rightfully be called cakes. Store-bought breads, even whole grain breads, sometimes reveal highly saturated fats like coconut oil, palm kernel oil, and cottonseed oil in their ingredients list. Store-bought coffee cakes are drenched in butter and other fats, and may contain more sugar than flour. Croissants are the worst, having twice as much fat as any comparable bagel or muffin—actually they should be considered a pastry. Homemade breads made with whole grains, vegetables, and fruits, like the ones in this chapter, are the real "staff of life."

A Primer on Leavening

Leavening agents are the ingredients that cause baked goods to rise to a pleasing light texture. "Quick breads" are raised by baking powder or baking soda; they can be baked as soon as they're mixed. Yeast breads take longer because they need time to rise.

Baking Soda

Also known as bicarbonate of soda, baking soda is an alkali. When you combine it with moisture and an acid such as sour milk, buttermilk, yogurt, molasses, or fruit juice, it produces bubbles of carbon dioxide gas that make the batter rise. It's fast acting, so the cook also has to act fast. As soon as you add the liquid ingredients to the dry, be prepared to mix the batter quickly, spoon it into a prepared pan, and bake it in a preheated oven at once.

Baking Powder

Single-acting baking powder is a combination of baking soda plus cream of tartar (a fruit acid) and a stabilizer such as cornstarch. Because it already contains the right combination to make carbon dioxide, it's okay not to have any acid ingredients in the batter. You can use sweet milk or whatever you wish. Since it's single-acting, batters made with this leavening must be baked promptly after mixing.

Double-acting baking powder, the kind sold in supermarkets today, contains two different acids so that it will react twice—first to moisture, when the liquid and dry ingredients are combined, and second to heat, when the bread or muffins are baked. That means the cook doesn't have to rush the pan into the oven. In a pinch, the batter can be refrigerated for several hours before baking. But if there's no reason to delay baking, don't.

In a pinch, the equivalent of 1 teaspoon single-acting baking powder can be improvised by mixing ½ teaspoon cream of tartar with ¼ teaspoon baking soda.

Yeast

Yeast is a living organism that needs a certain amount of babying. Warmth, moisture, and nourishment (flour and/or sugar) bring it to life. It multiplies and gives off carbon dioxide gas, which makes dough rise. Cold or drying retard the growth of yeast. Really hot temperatures kill it. When you bake with yeast, the yeast is killed but the raised structure of the dough remains. Kneading is required in many yeast recipes to strengthen the gluten in the flour so that the bread will hold its risen shape.

Most cooks these days are using active dry yeast, a granular form in which the yeast is temporarily deactivated by drying. Supermarkets sell this yeast in packets, each containing about 2½ teaspoons or 1 scant tablespoon. These convenient packets have a use-by date printed right on the envelope. They can be kept at room temperature, but keeping them in the refrigerator is a better policy. Best of all, put them into the freezer and they will keep indefinitely.

Active dry yeast should be dissolved in warm water before using, in whatever amount the recipe calls for. If you want to "proof" yeast (find out if it's truly active), add a teaspoon of sugar to the warm water and wait 5 minutes. The yeast should bubble up. Proofing is a simple insurance to make certain your yeast is still full of pep.

Instant active dry yeast is dried at a lower temperature; its granules are smaller and it doesn't need dissolving or "proofing." It can be added to dry ingredients before liquids are added, but the water must be very hot (125 to 130 degrees F) to activate it. It's sold in specialty baking supply stores. *Quick-rising* active dry yeast, sold in packets in the supermarket, may be treated like instant yeast. Your bread will develop a better flavor, however, if you take time to let it rise slowly.

Easy Whole Wheat Dinner Rolls

MAKES 16 TO 18 ROLLS

Just one rising makes these rolls a cinch to prepare.

1 (2½-teaspoon) package active
  dry yeast
1 teaspoon granulated sugar
1 cup plus 2 tablespoons
  warm water

3 cups whole wheat flour
½ cup nonfat dry milk powder
1 teaspoon salt
3 tablespoons brown sugar
2 tablespoons vegetable oil

Stir the yeast and granulated sugar into the warm water. Let stand for 5 minutes. It should bubble up and look active.

In the large bowl of an electric mixer, mix the flour, dry milk, salt, and brown sugar. With the motor running on low, mix in the oil. Add the yeast mixture and beat on medium speed until well combined. Alternatively, do the mixing by hand. If necessary to make the dough hold together, add a little more warm water, 1 tablespoon at a time.

With an electric dough hook, knead the dough for 5 minutes. Or transfer the dough to a floured board and knead by hand until it's smooth and not too sticky to handle, 8 to 10 minutes.

Spray two 9-inch pie pans with cooking spray. Divide the dough in half and roll into two 12-inch ropes. Cut each rope into 8 or 9 pieces. Place the pieces in the prepared pans, with one piece in the center, and let them rise in a warm place until they are well doubled, about 1½ hours.

Preheat the oven to 400 degrees F. Bake the rolls in the middle of the oven for about 15 minutes, until they are nicely browned top and bottom (raise them with a spatula to see the bottoms). Remove them from the pan to wire racks. If serving immediately, cool slightly to serve warm. If not, cool completely. Store in a plastic container or bag.

Kilocalories 106 Kc • Protein 3 gm • Fat 2 gm • Percent of calories from fat 17% • Cholesterol 0 mg • Dietary fiber 3 gm • Sodium 152 mg • Calcium 20 mg

CHEESE 'N WHEAT ROLLS: Follow the preceding recipe, reducing the salt to ¾ teaspoon. Add 1 cup coarsely grated longhorn cheese with the oil.

Kilocalories 126 Kc • Protein 5 gm • Fat 3 gm • Percent of calories from fat 23% • Cholesterol 5 mg • Dietary fiber 3 gm • Sodium 151 mg • Calcium 70 mg

ONION-WHEAT ROLLS: Follow the basic whole wheat dinner rolls recipe, adding 1 cup chopped sweet onion with the oil.

Kilocalories 110 Kc • Protein 4 gm • Fat 2 gm • Percent of calories from fat 17% • Cholesterol 0 mg • Dietary fiber 3 gm • Sodium 152 mg • Calcium 22 mg

WHOLE WHEAT SWEET BREAKFAST ROLLS: Follow the basic recipe for whole wheat dinner rolls, increasing the brown sugar to ¼ cup. In a bowl, mix together an additional ¼ cup brown sugar, ⅓ cup chopped unsalted pecans, ½ cup plumped raisins (see Note), and 1 teaspoon ground cinnamon.

After kneading, instead of making ropes of dough, roll the dough out into a 16 × 12-inch square and sprinkle it with the sugar-nut-raisin mixture. Roll up the dough like a jelly roll, press the ends to seal them, and stretch the roll out to 24 inches. Cut the roll into 16 pieces.

Preheat the oven to 375 degrees F. Continue as in the basic recipe.

NOTE: To plump raisins, soak them in very hot water for 5 minutes; drain well.

Kilocalories 151 Kc • Protein 4 gm • Fat 4 gm • Percent of calories from fat 20% • Cholesterol 0 mg • Dietary fiber 3 gm • Sodium 154 mg • Calcium 27 mg

Whole Wheat Potato Bread

MAKES 2 LOAVES

This is a moist loaf with a pleasing mild flavor—even if whole grain breads are not a favorite at your house, I think this one will make a hit.

1 small potato, peeled and diced (¼ pound)
½ cup brown sugar
2 (2½-teaspoon) packages dry yeast
3 cups whole wheat flour

3 cups unbleached all-purpose flour, plus ½ cup more if needed
1 teaspoon ground cardamom
1½ teaspoons salt
¼ cup vegetable oil

Put the potato in a small saucepan with 1 cup of water. Bring to a boil and cook until quite tender, about 8 minutes. Drain, reserving the water. Put the water into a 2-cup measuring cup and add enough tepid water to make 2 cups. Test the water; it should be warm but not hot. Stir 1 tablespoon brown sugar and the yeast into the water.

Mash the potato. When the yeast mixture is bubbly, combine it with the potato and the remaining brown sugar in the large bowl of an electric mixer. In another bowl, mix the whole wheat and white flours with the cardamom and salt. Spoon half of this into the yeast and beat with an electric mixer for 1 minute. Add the oil and continue to beat for 1 to 2 minutes, until the oil is well incorporated and the batter is smooth. Add the remaining flour.

With a dough hook (5 minutes) or by hand (10 minutes), knead the dough until it's a smooth ball. You may have to add another ½ cup flour. Put the dough in an oiled bowl and turn to coat all sides. Cover with plastic wrap and let rise in a warm place until doubled, 1 to 1½ hours.

Punch the dough down and shape it into 2 loaves. Put the loaves in 2 oiled 9 × 5-inch loaf pans and let the dough rise until it reaches the top of the pans, 1 to 1½ hours.

Preheat the oven to 375 degrees F. Bake the loaves in the middle of the oven for 30 minutes, or until the bottoms sound hollow when tapped. (Raise one of the breads from the pan with a spatula to check.) Remove from the pans and cool completely on wire racks before slicing.

Kilocalories 146 Kc • Protein 4 gm • Fat 3 gm • Percent of calories from fat 16% • Cholesterol 0 mg • Dietary fiber 2 gm • Sodium 149 mg • Calcium 12 mg

WHOLE WHEAT RAISIN BREAD: Follow the preceding recipe, substituting ground cinnamon for the cardamom. Blend in 1½ cups plumped raisins (see Note, page 269) with the second addition of flour.

Kilocalories 173 Kc • Protein 4 gm • Fat 3 gm • Percent of calories from fat 14% • Cholesterol 0 mg • Dietary fiber 3 gm • Sodium 150 mg • Calcium 17 mg

WHOLE WHEAT FRUIT 'N NUT BREAD: Follow the basic whole wheat bread recipe. Blend in 1 cup coarsely chopped unsalted walnuts, ½ cup chopped dried apricots, and ½ cup sweetened dried cranberries with the second addition of flour.

Kilocalories 192 Kc • Protein 5 gm • Fat 6 gm • Percent of calories from fat 25% • Cholesterol 0 mg • Dietary fiber 3 gm • Sodium 149 mg • Calcium 17 mg

Spiced Carrot Brown Bread

---■---

MAKES 2 BREADS

A traditional brown soda bread gets a nice slice of beta-carotene. The extra bread can be wrapped in foil and frozen.

½ cup nonfat plain yogurt
½ cup low-fat milk
2 cups whole wheat flour
2 cups unbleached all-
  purpose flour
1 tablespoon baking soda
½ teaspoon salt
2 teaspoons ground cinnamon
½ teaspoon ground nutmeg

½ teaspoon ground allspice
⅓ cup brown sugar
1 cup plumped golden raisins
  (see Note, page 269)
1 cup finely grated carrots
  (about 3)
¼ cup canola oil
Additional milk or flour if
  needed

Preheat the oven to 350 degrees F. Spray 2 round 8- to 9-inch pans, such as cake pans, with cooking spray.

In a small pitcher, mix the yogurt and milk. In a large bowl, sift together the flours, baking soda, salt, and spices. Blend in the brown sugar, raisins, and carrots. Add the canola oil and yogurt mixture. As necessary, add a little more milk or a spoonful of flour to make a soft but manageable dough. Knead the dough briefly, just enough to smooth it, then form it into 2 round loaves. Place them in the prepared pans. Gently cut an inch-deep cross in the top of each.

Bake in the middle of the oven until they are nicely browned and a wooden pick or cake tester inserted in the centers comes out dry, about 35 minutes. If the tops brown too quickly, lay a sheet of foil over them until they finish cooking. Remove the breads from the pans and cool them on wire racks before slicing.

Kilocalories 194 Kc • Protein 5 gm • Fat 4 gm • Percent of calories from fat 19% • Cholesterol 1 mg • Dietary fiber 3 gm • Sodium 324 mg • Calcium 48 mg

Bell Pepper Corn Bread

The best pan for this bread is a cast-iron frying pan, which will give it a golden, crispy bottom crust.

4 tablespoons vegetable oil
1 red bell pepper, seeded
   and diced
1 green bell pepper, seeded
   and diced
2 scallions, chopped
¼ teaspoon dried thyme
1 cup unbleached all-
   purpose flour

1 tablespoon baking powder
2 teaspoons sugar
½ teaspoon salt
1 cup cornmeal (preferably
   whole grain)
1 cup low-fat milk
1 egg

Preheat the oven to 400 degrees F.

Heat 1 tablespoon of oil in a 10-inch cast-iron frying pan (or any heavy skillet with a flameproof handle), and slowly sauté the peppers and scallions until they are tender but not brown, 5 minutes. Remove from the heat and stir in the thyme.

Sift together the flour, baking powder, sugar, and salt. Stir in the cornmeal. In a bowl, beat together the milk, egg, and remaining 3 tablespoons of oil. Pour the liquid ingredients into the dry and stir until blended. Fold the batter into the bell-pepper mixture in the frying pan.

Bake the bread in the top third of the oven until golden on top and dry inside when tested with a wooden pick or cake tester, 18 to 20 minutes. Serve warm, cut into wedges. Remove leftovers from the pan. When completely cool, wrap in foil and refrigerate or freeze.

Kilocalories 203 Kc • Protein 5 gm • Fat 9 gm • Percent of calories from fat 39% • Cholesterol 29 mg • Dietary fiber 2 gm • Sodium 325 mg • Calcium 107 mg

Sweet Potato Corn Bread

---◼---

Sweet potato adds a bonus of antioxidants to this down-home corn bread.

About 1 teaspoon soft unsalted butter

1 small sweet potato, peeled and diced (½ pound)

1½ cups unbleached all-purpose flour

¼ cup sugar

1 teaspoon baking powder

½ teaspoon baking soda

1 teaspoon ground allspice

½ teaspoon salt

1 cup whole grain cornmeal

1 egg

½ cup low-fat milk

½ cup nonfat plain yogurt

2 tablespoons vegetable oil

Preheat the oven to 400 degrees F. Melt the butter in a 10-inch cast-iron frying pan or a 9 × 9-inch baking pan. Coat the sides as well as the bottom of the pan with the butter.

Boil or steam the sweet potato until tender, 10 to 15 minutes. Drain well and mash the potato. You should have 1 cup.

Sift together the flour, sugar, baking powder, baking soda, allspice, and salt. Stir in the cornmeal. In another bowl, beat together the egg, milk, yogurt, sweet potato, and oil. Pour the liquid ingredients into the dry and stir until blended. Spoon the batter into the prepared pan and smooth the top with a spatula (the batter will be thick).

Bake the bread in the top third of the oven until golden on top and dry inside when tested with a wooden pick or cake tester, 18 to 20 minutes. Serve warm, cut into wedges. Remove leftovers from the pan.

Kilocalories 238 Kc • Protein 5 gm • Fat 5 gm • Percent of calories from fat 18% • Cholesterol 3 mg • Dietary fiber 3 gm • Sodium 301 mg • Calcium 80 mg

Quick, Savory Scallion Bread

This is just the bread to fill out a soup supper in style. It's made as easily as corn bread, using whole wheat instead.

4 tablespoons vegetable oil
1 bunch scallions, chopped
1 cup whole wheat flour
1 cup unbleached all-
   purpose flour
1 teaspoon baking powder
½ teaspoon baking soda

2 teaspoons sugar
½ teaspoon salt
¼ teaspoon dried rosemary
¾ cup nonfat plain yogurt
½ cup low-fat milk
1 egg

Preheat the oven to 400 degrees F.

Heat 1 tablespoon of the oil in a 10-inch cast-iron frying pan (or any heavy skillet with a flameproof handle) and slowly sauté the scallions until they are tender but not brown, 5 minutes. Remove from the heat.

Sift together the flours, baking powder, baking soda, sugar, and salt. Stir in the rosemary. Beat together the yogurt, milk, egg, and remaining 3 tablespoons of oil. Pour the liquid ingredients into the dry and stir until blended. Fold the batter into the scallion mixture in the frying pan.

Bake the bread in the top third of the oven until golden on top and dry inside when tested with a wooden pick or cake tester, 18 to 20 minutes. Serve warm, cut into wedges. Remove leftovers from the pan. When completely cool, wrap in foil and refrigerate or freeze.

Kilocalories 194 Kc • Protein 6 gm • Fat 8 gm • Percent of calories from fat 37% • Cholesterol 28 mg • Dietary fiber 2 gm • Sodium 302 mg • Calcium 81 mg

BREADS AND MUFFINS

Whole Grain Pineapple Bread

■

MAKES 8 SERVINGS

This really quick and easy bread can be served for brunch or with after-noon tea or coffee.

1 cup whole wheat flour
1 cup unbleached all-
  purpose flour
¼ cup sugar
1 teaspoon baking powder
½ teaspoon baking soda

¼ teaspoon salt
1 egg
½ cup low-fat milk
¼ cup vegetable oil
1 (8-ounce) can crushed
  pineapple, undrained

Preheat the oven to 400 degrees F. Butter and flour a 9 × 9-inch baking pan.

In a medium bowl, sift together the flours, sugar, baking powder, baking soda, and salt. In another bowl, mix the egg, milk, and oil. Stir in the undrained pineapple.

Pour the pineapple mixture into the dry ingredients and mix until smooth. Spoon the batter into the prepared pan.

Bake in the top third of the oven until a wooden pick or cake tester inserted in the center comes out dry, about 25 minutes.

Kilocalories 215 Kc • Protein 5 gm • Fat 8 gm • Percent of calories from fat 33% • Cholesterol 28 mg • Dietary fiber 2 gm • Sodium 218 mg • Calcium 54 mg

PINEAPPLE-PECAN BREAD: Follow the preceding recipe. After mixing the batter, fold in ½ cup pecan halves.

Kilocalories 259 Kc • Protein 5 gm • Fat 13 gm • Percent of calories from fat 43% • Cholesterol 28 mg • Dietary fiber 3 gm • Sodium 218 mg • Calcium 56 mg

Cranberry Nugget-Pumpkin Bread

You won't really believe this works unless you try it. The cranberry sauce does not dissolve into the bread but remains intact in tasty nuggets throughout. Making two breads uses all of the canned pumpkin and cranberry sauce—no worrisome leftovers!

3¾ cups unbleached all-purpose flour
2 teaspoons baking soda
2 teaspoon baking powder
2 teaspoons ground ginger
2 teaspoons ground cinnamon
½ teaspoon ground cloves
½ teaspoon salt
1 (15-ounce) can solid pack pumpkin

1¼ cups sugar
¼ cup wheat germ (or increase flour ¼ cup)
3 eggs, beaten
¾ cup canola oil
½ cup nonfat plain yogurt
1 (16-ounce) can jellied cranberry sauce (not whole berry), diced (see Note)

Preheat the oven to 350 degrees F. Spray 2 loaf pans with cooking spray. Line the bottoms with plain wax paper and spray that also. (Alternatively, use butter and flour.)

Sift the flour, baking soda, baking powder, spices, and salt into a large bowl. In a separate bowl or in a food processor, blend the pumpkin, sugar, wheat germ, eggs, oil, and yogurt. Beat the pumpkin mixture into the dry ingredients. *Gently* fold the diced cranberry sauce into the batter. Divide the batter between the 2 prepared pans.

Bake in the middle of the oven for 45 to 50 minutes, or until the breads have risen, browned, and shrunk slightly from the sides of the pan. A cake tester inserted in the centers should come out dry.

Cool the breads on wire racks for 10 minutes before turning out of the pans to cool completely. Handle them carefully; they are delicate until they cool. Strip off the wax paper. When completely cool, wrap in foil and refrigerate. The extra bread freezes well.

NOTE: To dice cranberry sauce, open both ends of the can, loosen the sides, and remove the sauce in one piece. Cut in half lengthwise, and then into long strips. Cut the strips into dice-size pieces.

Oatmeal-Fruit Muffins

◼

MAKES 12 MUFFINS

You can save time in baking breakfast muffins by sifting the dry ingredients and mixing the liquid ingredients the night before. Refrigerate the liquid mixture. The next morning, when the oven is hot and you're ready to bake, quickly mix the liquid and dry ingredients.

1 cup unbleached all-purpose flour	½ cup well-packed brown sugar
⅞ cup (1 cup minus 2 tablespoons) whole wheat flour	¾ cup low-fat milk
	1 large whole egg
1 tablespoon baking powder	1 egg white
1 teaspoon ground cinnamon	⅓ cup vegetable oil
½ teaspoon salt	½ cup chopped dried apricots
1 cup quick-cooking oats	¼ cup golden raisins, plumped (see Note, page 269)

Preheat the oven to 400 degrees F.

Spray a nonstick 12-cup muffin tin with cooking spray or use paper liners.

Sift together the flours, baking powder, cinnamon, and salt. Stir in the oats and brown sugar. In a separate bowl, whisk together the milk, egg, egg white, and oil. Beat the liquid ingredients into the dry ingredients until blended. Fold in the apricots and raisins.

Divide the batter between the muffin cups. Bake in the top third of the oven until the muffins are risen, lightly browned, and dry inside when tested with a wooden pick or cake tester, 15 to 20 minutes.

As soon as they can be handled, remove the muffins to a wire rack. Cool slightly. Serve warm.

Kilocalories 217 Kc • Protein 5 gm • Fat 7 gm • Percent of calories from fat 30% • Cholesterol 19 mg • Dietary fiber 3 gm • Sodium 220 mg • Calcium 83 mg

Whole Grain Blueberry Muffins

I make lots of these wonderful breakfast treats when blueberries are in season. The muffins will keep two to three days in a plastic container in the refrigerator.

1 cup low-fat milk
1 tablespoon white vinegar
½ cup sugar
1 teaspoon ground cinnamon
1¼ cups unbleached all-purpose flour
1 cup plus 2 tablespoons whole wheat flour

2 teaspoons baking soda
½ teaspoon salt
2 large eggs or ½ cup egg substitute, such as Egg Beaters
⅓ cup vegetable oil
1 heaping cup fresh or frozen blueberries, preferably small blueberries

Preheat the oven to 400 degrees F. Spray a 12-cup nonstick muffin pan with cooking spray or use paper liners.

Mix together the milk and vinegar, and let the mixture stand for 10 to 15 minutes at room temperature to sour the milk. In a small bowl, mix together 1 teaspoon of the sugar with ¼ teaspoon of the cinnamon; reserve for sprinkling on the muffins.

Sift together the flours, remaining sugar, baking soda, salt, and remaining ¾ teaspoon cinnamon into a large bowl. Beat together the soured milk, eggs, and oil. Pour the liquid ingredients into the dry ingredients and stir to blend. Fold in the blueberries.

Divide the batter between the muffin cups and sprinkle with the cinnamon-sugar mixture. Bake in the top third of the oven for 18 to 20 minutes, until the muffins are risen, lightly browned, and a cake tester inserted in the center comes out dry.

As soon as the muffins can be handled, remove them from the pan to a wire rack. Serve warm or at room temperature.

Kilocalories 197 Kc • Protein 5 gm • Fat 8 gm • Percent of calories from fat 34% • Cholesterol 37 mg • Dietary fiber 2 gm • Sodium 329 mg • Calcium 38 mg

BREADS AND MUFFINS

PEACH-GINGER MUFFINS: Follow the preceding recipe. Substitute ground ginger for the cinnamon and ¼ cup diced peeled fresh or canned peaches, well drained, for the blueberries.

Kilocalories 192 Kc • Protein 5 gm • Fat 8 gm • Percent of calories from fat 35% • Cholesterol 37 mg • Dietary fiber 2 gm • Sodium 328 mg • Calcium 35 mg

Apple-Carrot Muffins

■

MAKES 12 MUFFINS

These are delicious with a salad for lunch or as an after-school snack.

½ cup sugar
½ teaspoon ground cinnamon
2½ cups unbleached all-
  purpose flour
2¼ teaspoons baking powder
¼ teaspoon ground cloves
¼ teaspoon ground allspice
½ teaspoon salt

1 cup low-fat milk
1 large whole egg
1 egg white
⅓ cup vegetable oil
1 cup finely diced peeled apple
  (1 medium)
1 cup coarsely grated carrot
  (2 small)

Preheat the oven to 400 degrees F. Spray a 12-cup nonstick muffin pan with cooking spray or use paper liners.

In a small bowl, mix together 1 teaspoon of the sugar with ¼ teaspoon of the cinnamon; reserve for sprinkling on the muffins.

Sift together the flour, remaining sugar, baking powder, cloves, all-spice, the remaining ¼ teaspoon cinnamon, and the salt into a large bowl. Beat together the milk, egg, egg white, and oil. Pour the liquid ingredients into the dry ingredients and stir to blend. Fold in the apple and carrot.

Divide the batter between the muffin cups and sprinkle them with the cinnamon-sugar mixture. Bake in the top third of the oven for 15 to 18 minutes, until the muffins are risen, lightly browned, and a cake tester inserted in the center comes out dry.

As soon as the muffins can be handled, remove them from the pan to a wire rack. Serve warm or at room temperature.

Orange Bran Muffins

MAKES **12** MUFFINS

Bran is rich in fiber and nerve-building B vitamins as well as antioxidant vitamin E.

2 cups unbleached all-
  purpose flour
1 teaspoon baking powder
½ teaspoon baking soda
½ teaspoon ground cinnamon
½ teaspoon salt
½ cup toasted bran (see Note)
½ cup well-packed brown sugar

1 cup orange juice
1 teaspoon grated orange zest
1 large whole egg
1 egg white
⅓ cup vegetable oil
½ cup raisins, plumped (see
  Note, page 269)

Preheat the oven to 400 degrees F.

Spray a nonstick 12-cup muffin tin with cooking spray or use paper liners.

Sift together the flour, baking powder, baking soda, cinnamon, and salt. Stir in the bran and brown sugar. In a separate bowl, whisk together the orange juice, orange zest, egg, egg white, and oil. Beat the liquid ingredients into the dry ingredients until blended. Fold in the raisins.

Divide the batter between the muffin cups. Bake in the top third of the oven until the muffins are risen, lightly browned, and dry inside when tested with a cake tester, 15 to 20 minutes.

As soon as they can be handled, remove the muffins to a wire rack. Cool slightly. Serve warm.

NOTE: Toasted bran is sold in jars in the cereal section of most supermarkets.

Pineapple-Pear Muffins

■

This is a nice muffin to serve with afternoon tea. This British custom has become a popular import, with many fine hotels serving a full English tea.

½ cup sugar

1 teaspoon ground ginger

1 (8-ounce) can crushed
  pineapple

About ¾ cup low-fat milk

2½ cups unbleached all-
  purpose flour

1 teaspoon baking powder

½ teaspoon baking soda

½ teaspoon salt

1 large whole egg

1 egg white

⅓ cup vegetable oil

1 cup finely diced peeled pear
  (1 large)

Preheat the oven to 400 degrees F. Spray a 12-cup nonstick muffin pan with cooking spray or use paper liners.

In a small bowl, mix together 1 teaspoon of the sugar with ¼ teaspoon of the ginger; reserve for sprinkling on the muffins. Drain the pineapple, reserving the juice. Pour the juice into a measuring cup and add enough milk to make 1 cup.

Sift together the flour, remaining sugar, baking powder, baking soda, the remaining ¾ teaspoon ginger, and the salt into a large bowl. Beat together the milk-juice mixture, egg, egg white, and oil. Pour the liquid ingredients into the dry ingredients and stir to blend. Fold in the pear and pineapple.

Divide the batter between the muffin cups and sprinkle them with the ginger-sugar mixture. Bake in the top third of the oven for 15 to 18 minutes, until the muffins are risen, lightly browned, and a cake tester inserted in the center comes out dry.

As soon as the muffins can be handled, remove them from the pan to a wire rack. Serve warm or at room temperature.

Kilocalories 206 Kc • Protein 4 gm • Fat 7 gm • Percent of calories from fat 31% • Cholesterol 19 mg • Dietary fiber 1 gm • Sodium 201 mg • Calcium 43 mg

ANTIOXIDANT POWER

Corn-Raspberry Muffins

A sweet, grainy corn muffin with the tart taste of raspberries makes a nice start to any morning!

1½ cups unbleached all-purpose flour
½ cup sugar
1 teaspoon baking powder
½ teaspoon baking soda
½ teaspoon ground cardamom
½ teaspoon salt
1 cup whole grain cornmeal

1 large whole egg
1 egg white
⅓ cup vegetable oil
1 cup nonfat plain yogurt
1 cup frozen unsweetened raspberries (separate but unthawed)

Preheat the oven to 400 degrees F.

Spray a nonstick 12-cup muffin tin with cooking spray or use paper liners.

Sift together the flour, sugar, baking powder, baking soda, cardamom, and salt. Stir in the cornmeal. In a separate bowl, whisk together the egg, egg white, oil, and yogurt. Beat the liquid ingredients into the dry ingredients until blended. Fold in the frozen raspberries.

Divide the batter between the muffin cups. Bake in the top third of the oven until the muffins are risen, lightly browned, and dry inside when tested with a cake tester, 15 to 20 minutes.

As soon as they can be handled, remove the muffins to a wire rack. Cool slightly. Serve warm.

Kilocalories 198 Kc • Protein 4 gm • Fat 7 gm • Percent of calories from fat 31% • Cholesterol 18 mg • Dietary fiber 1 gm • Sodium 211 mg • Calcium 56 mg

Pumpkin-Pecan Biscuits

MAKES ABOUT 12 BISCUITS

This is a reduced-fat, antioxidant-enriched version of that old-time standby, baking powder biscuits.

2½ cups unbleached all-
  purpose flour
2 tablespoons brown sugar
1 tablespoon baking powder
½ teaspoon salt
½ teaspoon ground cinnamon
¼ teaspoon ground nutmeg
2 tablespoons unsalted butter

½ cup canola oil
¾ cup mashed unflavored
  canned or fresh cooked
  pumpkin
2 tablespoons chopped unsalted
  pecans
About ½ cup low-fat milk

Preheat the oven to 400 degrees F. Spray a baking sheet with cooking spray.

Sift together the flour, brown sugar, baking powder, salt, cinnamon, and nutmeg. With a pastry cutter or 2 knives, cut in the butter until the mixture is mealy. Whisk together the oil and pumpkin, and stir it into the flour mixture. Stir in the pecans. Add enough milk to make a soft dough.

Transfer the dough to a floured surface and knead it gently until it can be patted into a ½-inch-thick round. With a floured biscuit cutter or glass, cut the biscuits and place them on the baking sheet, rerolling the scraps.

Bake the biscuits in the top of the oven for about 12 minutes, or until they are lightly browned and firm. Serve warm.

Kilocalories 203 Kc • Protein 3 gm • Fat 12 gm • Percent of calories from fat 50% • Cholesterol 3 mg • Dietary fiber 1 gm • Sodium 205 mg • Calcium 70 mg

Banana-Mango Coffee Cake

The use of pureed fruits makes it possible to use less fat in baked goods.

1 teaspoon unsalted butter,
    softened
1 cup unbleached all-
    purpose flour
1 cup whole wheat flour
½ cup sugar
1 teaspoon baking soda
½ teaspoon ground ginger
¼ teaspoon salt

1 large whole egg
1 egg white
¼ cup vegetable oil
¼ cup orange juice
1 cup pureed banana (from
    2 medium to small bananas)
1 cup diced ripe mango, well
    drained (½ mango)

Preheat the oven to 350 degrees F. Use the soft butter to grease a 9-inch square baking pan; this will give a nice buttery taste to the crust, even though there's no butter in the coffee cake.

Sift the flours, sugar, baking soda, ginger, and salt into a large bowl. In a separate bowl, whisk the egg, egg white, oil, and juice together. Blend in the pureed banana. Beat the liquid ingredients into the dry ingredients, and fold in the mango. Spoon the batter into the prepared pan.

Bake in the middle of the oven until a cake tester inserted in the center comes out dry, about 35 minutes. Let the cake cool slightly. Cut in squares and serve warm from the pan.

Kilocalories 353 Kc • Protein 7 gm • Fat 11 gm • Percent of calories from fat 27% • Cholesterol 36 mg • Dietary fiber 4 gm • Sodium 329 mg • Calcium 20 mg

Upside-Down Apricot Coffee Cake

———————————— ◼ ————————————

MAKES 6 SERVINGS

Beta-carotene-rich fresh apricots may be available only in June and July, but apricots canned in fruit juice are an equally nutritious substitute.

2 tablespoons unsalted butter
⅓ cup brown sugar
8 to 10 small ripe fresh
   apricots, unpeeled, halved, or
   1 (30-ounce) can apricots in
   juice pack, well drained
About ⅓ cup whole blanched
   almonds

1 cup plus 2 tablespoons
   unbleached all-purpose flour
1½ teaspoons baking powder
¼ teaspoon salt
3 eggs
⅓ cup granulated sugar
1 teaspoon natural almond
   flavoring

Preheat the oven to 350 degrees F.

Melt the butter over direct heat in a 9- to 10-inch skillet with a flame-proof handle, such as a cast-iron frying pan. Remove from the heat, add the brown sugar, and mix thoroughly. Spread the sugar evenly over the bottom. Arrange the apricot halves, cut sides up, over the sugar. (You may have a few left over. They'll make a nice dessert on another day.) Tuck the almonds between the apricots.

Stir together the flour, baking powder, and salt. Beat the eggs until they're light and fluffy. Gradually add the granulated sugar. Beat in the almond flavoring. Add the dry ingredients and beat until well blended. Pour the batter carefully over the apricots. The batter will be a thin cover; spread it evenly with a spatula.

Bake in the middle of the oven until a cake tester inserted in the center comes out clean, about 25 minutes. Remove the coffee cake from the oven and let it stand on a wire rack for 10 minutes. Loosen the edges and invert onto a serving plate. Serve warm.

Kilocalories 290 Kc • Protein 8 gm • Fat 9 gm • Percent of calories from fat 27% • Cholesterol 111 mg • Dietary fiber 3 gm • Sodium 237 mg • Calcium 92 mg

Whole Grain Streusel Coffee Bread

MAKES **8** SERVINGS

For a gala presentation, fill the center of the bread and garnish the sides with fresh berries.

½ cup chopped unsalted pecans
⅓ cup brown sugar
1 teaspoon ground cinnamon
1 cup whole wheat flour
1 cup unbleached all-
   purpose flour
¾ cup granulated sugar
2 teaspoons baking powder
½ teaspoon baking soda

¼ teaspoon salt
½ cup whole grain cornmeal
2 large eggs, beaten
½ cup nonfat plain yogurt
½ cup low-fat milk
½ cup vegetable oil
2 teaspoons vanilla extract
½ cup raisins, plumped (see
   Note, page 269)

Preheat the oven to 350 degrees F. Spray a tube pan with a removable rim with cooking spray or butter and flour it.

Mix together the pecans, brown sugar, and cinnamon.

Sift together the flours, granulated sugar, baking powder, baking soda, and salt. Stir in the cornmeal. In the large bowl of an electric mixer (or any large bowl for hand mixing), beat together the eggs, yogurt, milk, oil, and vanilla. Add the flour mixture and beat until blended. Stir in the raisins.

Spoon half the batter into the prepared pan. Sprinkle with half the pecan mixture. Spread the remaining batter on top. Sprinkle with the remaining pecan mixture. Bake in the middle of the oven until a cake tester inserted in the center comes out dry, about 35 minutes. Cool in the pan on a wire rack for 5 minutes. Remove the rim. When the bread is only slightly warm, remove it from the rest of the pan.

Kilocalories 469 Kc • Protein 8 gm • Fat 20 gm • Percent of calories from fat 38% • Cholesterol 54 mg • Dietary fiber 4 gm • Sodium 294 mg • Calcium 119 mg

Salads

In American culinary history, no dish has changed more than the salad. It has run the gamut from sweet to savory, from gelled to leafy, from cold to warm, and from composed to casual—depending on the fashions of the moment. But no matter what the current food stylists propose, salads have always provided us with a variety of antioxidants in one tasty dish, and they are liable to continue in that tradition.

Raw foods in salads provide an even more potent and fresher supply of antioxidants than cooked dishes. There are a few vegetables, however, that are just as nutrient-rich when cooked—but not overcooked. The beta-carotene in carrots, for instance, is made more available to the body when they are cooked. On the other hand, the vitamin C content of any vegetable is higher when eaten raw. In any case, a salad usually combines several antioxidant foods in their near-to-natural state and includes the bonus of salad oil, one of the best sources of vitamin E. A big helping of salad once a day will go a long way toward fulfilling your daily requirement for antioxidants.

Most salads include some kind of leafy greens. It's important to wash these well, even headed greens like iceberg lettuce, to remove sand, pesticides and whatever else may be clinging to them. Two or three dunks in cool water should do it. For curly-leaf greens that hang onto grit, such as escarole or chicory, it's even better to hold each leaf under running water for a few seconds as a finishing step. Even bagged greens that say "washed" on the package should be rinsed again in your own kitchen. The next step, of course, is to spin dry the greens or dry them by wrapping in kitchen towels so that the salad won't be soggy.

While making a tossed green salad is easy work, it does seem to take a lot of kitchen space when the washing, spinning dry, slicing, and dicing is going on. If you like to get this type of salad made ahead of time (and out of the way) without having it go limp, try this method: Pour the dressing into the bottom of the salad bowl, add any ingredients that improve when marinated, such as onion or cabbage, and stir them into the dressing. Then put on top those ingredients that need to remain crisp, such as lettuce or carrot curls, *and don't toss the salad.* Chill the salad (if that's what the directions dictate), and toss just before serving for a crisp, fresh dish. The onion will be sweeter, too.

The balance of a hot meal is always improved by the addition of something cold with a contrasting texture. So for balance and for health's sake, a salad is the ideal accompaniment to the main meal. It also makes a splendid lunch all on its own. So crunch away!

Tossed Green Salad

MAKES 4 SERVINGS

No tomato-sauced pasta dish should be served without a salad like this on the same menu.

¼ cup extra-virgin or regular
  olive oil
2 tablespoons red wine vinegar
¼ teaspoon salt
Freshly ground black pepper
2 inner celery stalks, sliced
4 scallions, chopped

2 cups stemmed tender young
  spinach leaves, chicory, or
  frisée, torn into bite-size pieces
½ head romaine lettuce or
  1 small head red leaf lettuce,
  torn into bite-size pieces

In a salad bowl, combine the oil, vinegar, and salt and pepper to taste. Toss with the celery and scallions. Put the leafy greens on top without tossing and chill until needed. Toss well just before serving.

Kilocalories 139 Kc • Protein 2 gm • Fat 14 gm • Percent of calories from fat 85% • Cholesterol 0 mg • Dietary fiber 2 gm • Sodium 190 mg • Calcium 60 mg

TOSSED GREENS WITH FENNEL: Follow the basic recipe, substituting 1 small cored chopped fennel bulb for the celery.

Kilocalories 143 Kc • Protein 2 gm • Fat 14 gm • Percent of calories from fat 82% • Cholesterol 0 mg • Dietary fiber 3 gm • Sodium 184 mg • Calcium 63 mg

TOSSED GREENS WITH OLIVES AND FETA CHEESE: Follow the basic recipe, topping the greens with 8 pitted halved kalamata olives and 2 ounces crumbled feta cheese. Omit the salt.

Kilocalories 197 Kc • Protein 4 gm • Fat 19 gm • Percent of calories from fat 82% • Cholesterol 12 mg • Dietary fiber 2 gm • Sodium 423 mg • Calcium 130 mg

TOSSED GREENS WITH GORGONZOLA: Follow the basic recipe, topping the greens with 2 ounces crumbled Gorgonzola cheese.

Kilocalories 189 Kc • Protein 5 gm • Fat 18 gm • Percent of calories from fat 82% • Cholesterol 11 mg • Dietary fiber 2 gm • Sodium 388 mg • Calcium 135 mg

TOSSED GREENS WITH RADICCHIO: Follow the basic recipe, substituting ½ small head of radicchio (¼ pound) for the celery.

Kilocalories 143 Kc • Protein 2 gm • Fat 14 gm • Percent of calories from fat 83% • Cholesterol 0 mg • Dietary fiber 2 gm • Sodium 179 mg • Calcium 58 mg

TOSSED GREENS WITH TOMATO AND CUCUMBER: Follow the basic recipe. Slice 1 large ripe tomato into wedges and marinate it with the celery and scallions at the bottom of the salad bowl. Peel and slice 1 small cucumber and layer it on top of the tomato. Top with the greens without tossing until ready to serve.

Kilocalories 159 Kc • Protein 3 gm • Fat 14 gm • Percent of calories from fat 75% • Cholesterol 0 mg • Dietary fiber 3 gm • Sodium 183 mg • Calcium 70 mg

Caesar Salad . . . by Way of Athens

Flavored with Kasseri, a firm sheep's milk cheese, and Greek olives, this Caesar salad is a tasty melding of two cuisines.

1 small head romaine, leaves broken into bite-size pieces
2 small ripe tomatoes, cut into wedges
½ cup loosely packed slivered Kasseri cheese

8 pitted kalamata olives, halved
½ cup Caesar Salad Dressing with Roasted Garlic (page 21), or more to your taste
1 cup Whole Wheat Croutons (page 311)

Put the lettuce in a large salad bowl. Arrange the tomatoes on top. Sprinkle with the Kasseri and olives. When ready to serve, pour the dressing on top. Add the croutons and toss well to blend.

Kilocalories 295 Kc • Protein 6 gm • Fat 26 gm • Percent of calories from fat 77% • Cholesterol 14 mg • Dietary fiber 2 gm • Sodium 363 mg • Calcium 125 mg

Sautéed Radicchio Salad

MAKES 4 SERVINGS

This is an enjoyable combination of textures and flavors.

1½ tablespoons olive oil
1 large yellow onion, sliced
1 garlic clove, chopped
1 head radicchio, cored and sliced (about ½ pound)
Salt and freshly ground black pepper

2 tablespoons red wine vinegar
4 cups shredded romaine lettuce (about ½ head)
About 4 teaspoons extra-virgin olive oil

Heat the oil in a large skillet, and sauté the onion and garlic for 1 minute. Add the radicchio and stir-fry until barely wilted, 3 minutes. Season with salt and pepper to taste. Toss with the vinegar. Cool.

Divide the romaine among 4 salad plates. Drizzle each portion with about 1 teaspoon extra-virgin olive oil. Divide the radicchio among the salads, heaping it on top of the romaine.

Kilocalories 123 Kc • Protein 2 gm • Fat 10 gm • Percent of calories from fat 69% • Cholesterol 0 mg • Dietary fiber 2 gm • Sodium 18 mg • Calcium 40 mg

Romaine, Watercress, Walnut, and Gorgonzola Salad

MAKES 4 SERVINGS

Not only are walnuts and walnut oil rich in vitamin E, this popular nut also yields the heart-healthy omega-3 fatty acids, usually only found in fish and flaxseed.

4 scallions with green tops, chopped
2 tablespoons red wine vinegar
2 tablespoons olive oil
1 tablespoon walnut oil
Freshly ground black pepper
½ head romaine, torn into bite-size pieces

1 large bunch watercress, tough stems removed, chopped
⅓ cup unsalted walnut halves or pieces, lightly toasted
2 ounces crumbled Gorgonzola cheese

In a large salad bowl, mix the scallions, vinegar, olive oil, and walnut oil with pepper to taste. (The cheese should supply enough salt.) Add the greens, but don't toss. Chill the salad. When ready to serve, sprinkle with the walnuts and cheese and toss well.

Kilocalories 217 Kc • Protein 7 gm • Fat 20 gm • Percent of calories from fat 80% • Cholesterol 11 mg • Dietary fiber 2 gm • Sodium 217 mg • Calcium 146 mg

Greens and Tomatoes with Avocado Dressing

MAKES 4 SERVINGS, ABOUT 1 CUP DRESSING

For a salad of mixed greens, choose two or more from romaine lettuce, red or green leafy lettuce, chicory, escarole (inner leaves), and watercress.

6 cups mixed greens, torn into
  bite-size pieces
4 large plum tomatoes, sliced
  into half rounds

2 scallions, chopped

For the dressing

1 ripe avocado, peeled and cut
  into chunks (about ⅓ pound)
¼ cup fresh lime juice (2 limes)
¼ cup olive oil

2 teaspoons sugar
½ teaspoon salt
⅛ to ¼ teaspoon white pepper

Baked tortilla chips as an
  accompaniment (optional)

Toss the greens, tomatoes, and scallions, and divide the salad among 4 plates.

For the dressing, combine all the ingredients in a food processor or blender and process until smooth. Stop the motor to scrape down the sides of the workbowl once or twice.

Divide the dressing among the salads or pass it separately. Garnish with tortilla chips, if desired.

Kilocalories 222 Kc • Protein 2 gm • Fat 21 gm • Percent of calories from fat 81% • Cholesterol 0 mg • Dietary fiber 4 gm • Sodium 304 mg • Calcium 43 mg

Sautéed Mushrooms and Watercress Salad

1 bunch watercress, stems removed, coarsely chopped

3 tablespoons olive oil

10 ounces baby Portobello mushrooms or any small brown mushrooms, cleaned, stems trimmed

1 red bell pepper, seeded and cut into thin strips

2 garlic cloves, minced

Salt and freshly ground black pepper

2 tablespoons balsamic vinegar

Arrange the watercress on a small platter and chill it.

Heat 2 tablespoons of oil in a 10-inch skillet, and stir-fry the mushrooms and pepper over medium-high heat until they begin to brown, about 5 minutes. Add the garlic, stir, lower the heat, and cook 1 minute longer. Season with salt and pepper to taste. Sprinkle with the vinegar. Let the mixture cool to room temperature.

When ready to serve, spoon the mushroom mixture over the watercress, leaving a border of green around the edge. Drizzle the remaining 1 tablespoon of oil over all.

Kilocalories 135 Kc • Protein 4 gm • Fat 10 gm • Percent of calories from fat 67% • Cholesterol 0 mg • Dietary fiber 3 gm • Sodium 24 mg • Calcium 79 mg

Watercress and Strawberry Salad

■

This pretty salad contrasts peppery greens with sweet-tart fruit—especially nice for a luncheon side dish.

1 bunch watercress, stems
   removed, coarsely chopped
4 cups red leaf lettuce, torn
   into bite-size pieces (about
   ½ head)
¼ cup olive oil

2 tablespoons or more raspberry
   vinegar
About ⅛ teaspoon freshly
   ground black pepper
2 cups halved small or quartered
   large strawberries

Combine the watercress and red leaf lettuce in a salad bowl; chill. Just before serving, toss with the oil, vinegar, and black pepper. Taste to determine if you want more vinegar. Add the strawberries and toss again gently.

Kilocalories 155 Kc • Protein 2 gm • Fat 14 gm • Percent of calories from fat 76% • Cholesterol 0 mg • Dietary fiber 3 gm • Sodium 20 mg • Calcium 89 mg

Spinach and Melon Salad

■

MAKES 4 SERVINGS

You need the mild flavor of young flat-leaf spinach for this salad, not the curly robust spinach sold in cellophane bags. Young spinach is often available when good ripe melons are also in season.

3 tablespoons raspberry vinegar
¼ teaspoon salt
3 tablespoons olive oil
2 cups cubed cantaloupe
2 cups cubed seedless
   watermelon

½ pound tender young spinach,
   washed, tough stems removed,
   and coarsely chopped
Fresh raspberries for garnish
   (optional)

In the bottom of a salad bowl, mix the vinegar with the salt until it's dissolved. Whisk in the oil. Taste the dressing. Add more salt or oil to taste. Stir in the melon cubes.

Add the spinach without tossing and chill the salad. When ready to serve, toss the salad, blending in the spinach. Garnish with fresh raspberries, if desired.

Kilocalories 157 Kc • Protein 3 gm • Fat 11 gm • Percent of calories from fat 58% • Cholesterol 0 mg • Dietary fiber 3 gm • Sodium 199 mg • Calcium 72 mg

Endive, Orange, and Walnut "Sunflower" Salad

■

MAKES 4 SERVINGS

Endive's slightly bitter flavor marries well with sweet oranges.

2 endives
4 outside romaine leaves, torn
   into large pieces
2 large navel oranges, peel and
   pith removed, sliced
½ cup walnut halves

2 tablespoons walnut oil
2 tablespoons orange juice
¼ teaspoon salt
1 teaspoon chopped fresh mint
   or ¼ teaspoon dried

Clean and core the endives. Keep the leaves whole. Make a bed of the romaine on a round plate. Add the endive leaves, arranged like flower petals. Overlap the orange slices at the center. Scatter the walnuts on top.

Whisk together the walnut oil, orange juice, salt, and mint. Drizzle the dressing over the salad. Let stand at room temperature for 15 minutes before serving.

Kilocalories 236 Kc • Protein 6 gm • Fat 16 gm • Percent of calories from fat 56% • Cholesterol 0 mg • Dietary fiber 7 gm • Sodium 151 mg • Calcium 88 mg

Red Grapefruit and Red Leaf Lettuce Salad

■

MAKES 4 SERVINGS

This salad is so refreshing, it's perfect to serve with one of the oily fish, such as swordfish.

2 red grapefruit	2 scallions, finely chopped
1 small head red-leaf lettuce	Salt and freshly ground black
3 tablespoons olive oil	pepper

Remove the peel and pith from the grapefruit. With a thin serrated knife, cut the grapefruit segments free of the encasing membrane, working over a bowl to catch the juices. Squeeze the membrane over the bowl before discarding it. Tear the lettuce into bite-size pieces.

Put the grapefruit in the bottom of a salad bowl. Add the olive oil, scallions, and 3 tablespoons of the reserved juice. (Save the remaining juice.) Season with salt and pepper to taste. Heap the lettuce on top and chill the salad without tossing. When ready to serve, toss the salad well and taste to determine if you want more oil, juice, salt, or pepper.

Kilocalories 137 Kc • Protein 1 gm • Fat 10 gm • Percent of calories from fat 65% • Cholesterol 0 mg • Dietary fiber 2 gm • Sodium 5 mg • Calcium 58 mg

Grapefruit, Papaya, and Romaine Salad

MAKES 4 SERVINGS

Along with its plentiful beta-carotene, papaya contains enzymes that enhance digestion.

1 large pink or white grapefruit	2 tablespoons rice vinegar
1 ripe papaya	¼ teaspoon salt
8 romaine lettuce leaves	1 teaspoon chopped fresh mint
3 tablespoons olive oil	

Remove the peel and pith from the grapefruit. With a thin serrated knife, cut the grapefruit segments free of the encasing membrane, working over a bowl to catch the juices. Squeeze the membrane over the bowl before discarding it.

Peel, seed, and cut the papaya into thin slices. Tear the lettuce into bite-size pieces.

Whisk together the oil, rice vinegar, salt, and 2 tablespoons of the grapefruit juice. Blend in the mint.

When ready to serve, place the lettuce in a salad bowl and drizzle with half the dressing. Arrange the papaya and grapefruit on top, and drizzle with the remaining dressing. Toss just before serving.

Kilocalories 178 Kc • Protein 1 gm • Fat 10 gm • Percent of calories from fat 52% • Cholesterol 0 mg • Dietary fiber 3 gm • Sodium 155 mg • Calcium 50 mg

Blood Orange and Red Onion Salad

―――――――――――――■―――――――――――――

MAKES 6 SERVINGS

This exotic version of a popular Sicilian salad can be doubled and is a colorful addition to a buffet. If you can't find blood oranges, use seeded temple oranges or navel oranges.

1 small red onion, peeled, sliced, and separated into rings

8 blood oranges, peel and pith removed, sliced

1 tablespoon minced fresh flat-leaf parsley

1 teaspoon chopped fresh mint leaves

2 tablespoons extra-virgin olive oil

Salt and freshly ground black pepper

Soak the onion rings in ice water to cover for a half hour or so. Drain well.

Arrange the sliced oranges on a platter. Scatter the onion rings on top. Sprinkle with parsley and mint. Drizzle on the olive oil, and season with salt and pepper to taste. Let stand for 20 minutes or more at room temperature before serving.

Kilocalories 130 Kc • Protein 2 gm • Fat 5 gm • Percent of calories from fat 31% • Cholesterol 0 mg • Dietary fiber 5 gm • Sodium 1 mg • Calcium 75 mg

Bibb Lettuce, Walnut, and Pear Salad

MAKES 4 SERVINGS

Toss this salad at the table after everyone has had a chance to admire it.

2 large ripe Bosc or Bartlett
    pears, peeled, cored, and sliced
    into thin wedges
3 tablespoons lemon juice
2 tablespoons olive oil
2 tablespoons walnut oil
½ teaspoon sugar

¼ teaspoon salt
⅛ teaspoon freshly ground black
    pepper
1 head Bibb lettuce, torn into
    bite-size pieces
½ cup unsalted walnut halves

Put the pears in a bowl of ice water to which you've added 1 tablespoon of the lemon juice.

Whisk together the olive oil, walnut oil, the remaining 2 tablespoons of lemon juice, the sugar, salt, and pepper.

Line a salad bowl with the greens. Just before serving, drain the pears well and arrange them in a fan on top. Sprinkle them with the walnuts and pour the dressing over all.

Kilocalories 267 Kc • Protein 5 gm • Fat 23 gm • Percent of calories from fat 72% • Cholesterol 0 mg • Dietary fiber 3 gm • Sodium 148 mg • Calcium 31 mg

Asparagus with Peanut Dressing

There's a spicy Asian influence in this appetizing asparagus salad.

**1 pound fresh asparagus, woody
ends removed, cut diagonally
into 2-inch pieces**

For the dressing

3 tablespoons rice vinegar
3 tablespoons peanut oil
**1 tablespoon naturally brewed
reduced-sodium soy sauce**
1 teaspoon sesame oil
**½ teaspoon hot pepper sauce,
such as Tabasco, or more,
to taste**

**½ teaspoon sugar (omit if rice
vinegar is seasoned)**
**¼ teaspoon salt (omit if rice
vinegar is seasoned)**
**1 slice fresh ginger, very finely
minced, or ½ teaspoon ground
ginger**
½ cup chopped unsalted peanuts

Lay the asparagus in a large skillet and add ¾ cup water. Bring to a boil and simmer, covered, until tender-crisp, 2 to 3 minutes. Drain and rinse in cold water; the easy way to do this is right in the skillet, using the pan cover to hold back the vegetable when you drain out the water. Chill the asparagus.

Whisk together all the dressing ingredients except the chopped peanuts. When ready to serve, toss the asparagus with the dressing. Sprinkle with the peanuts.

Kilocalories 222 Kc • Protein 7 gm • Fat 19 gm • Percent of calories from fat 76% • Cholesterol 0 mg • Dietary fiber 1 gm • Sodium 315 mg • Calcium 22 mg

BROCCOLI WITH WALNUT DRESSING: Follow the preceding recipe, substituting 1 pound broccoli crowns for the asparagus. Cut the stalks ½-inch thick with florets attached. Substitute walnut oil for peanut oil and unsalted walnut halves for peanuts.

Kilocalories 238 Kc • Protein 7 gm • Fat 21 gm • Percent of calories from fat 73% • Cholesterol 0 mg • Dietary fiber 4 gm • Sodium 331 mg • Calcium 66 mg

ANTIOXIDANT POWER

Green Bean, Tomato, and Mozzarella Salad

Try this attractive and popular salad as a buffet dish—but make a lot! The recipe can be doubled, tripled, or whatever you need.

¾ pound fresh green beans, ends trimmed

2 medium tomatoes, sliced into thin wedges

3 tablespoons extra-virgin olive oil

Kosher salt and freshly ground black pepper

1 garlic clove, crushed through a press

8 fresh basil leaves, slivered

2 to 4 ounces fresh mozzarella, diced

Cook the beans in boiling salted water until tender-crisp, 5 to 6 minutes. Immediately drain and rinse in cold water.

Put the tomatoes in a large salad bowl, and dress the slices with the oil, salt and pepper to taste, and the garlic, taking care to distribute it well throughout. Stir in the basil leaves and mozzarella. Let this mixture marinate at room temperature for 20 to 30 minutes. Stir in the green beans and continue to marinate, stirring occasionally, for 5 to 10 minutes before serving.

Kilocalories 163 Kc • Protein 7 gm • Fat 12 gm • Percent of calories from fat 59% • Cholesterol 4 mg • Dietary fiber 3 gm • Sodium 43 mg • Calcium 149 mg

Green Bean and Radicchio Salad

MAKES 4 SERVINGS

Use extra-virgin olive oil where the flavor really counts, such as in salads. For cooked dishes or sautéing, ordinary pure olive oil is fine.

½ pound fresh green beans, ends trimmed, cut diagonally into 2-inch pieces

3 tablespoons extra-virgin olive oil

2 tablespoons red wine vinegar

Salt and freshly ground black pepper

½ cup chopped Vidalia onion or any sweet onion

4 fresh basil leaves, chopped

1 small head radicchio, shredded (½ pound)

8 romaine lettuce leaves, torn into bite-size pieces

Cook the beans in boiling salted water until tender-crisp, 5 to 6 minutes. Immediately drain and rinse in cold water.

In a large salad bowl, combine the oil and vinegar with salt and pepper to taste. Stir in the onion and basil. Top with the green beans, radicchio, and romaine without stirring. Chill. When ready to serve, toss the salad well. Taste to see if you want more oil or vinegar.

Kilocalories 134 Kc • Protein 3 gm • Fat 11 gm • Percent of calories from fat 66% • Cholesterol 0 mg • Dietary fiber 3 gm • Sodium 17 mg • Calcium 52 mg

Green Bean and Fennel Salad

Fennel and apple complement each other nicely.

½ pound fresh green beans,
   ends trimmed, cut diagonally
   into 2-inch pieces
1 small fennel bulb, cored and
   chopped
1 unpeeled Granny Smith apple,
   cored and diced

2 teaspoons olive oil
8 romaine lettuce leaves, torn
   into bite-size pieces
4 scallions, chopped
1 large carrot, coarsely grated
⅓ cup Garlic and Lemon
   Vinaigrette (page 19)

Cook the beans in boiling salted water until tender-crisp, 5 to 6 minutes. Immediately drain and rinse in cold water.

Mix the fennel and apple with the olive oil, coating all sides, to prevent them from turning brown. Put the lettuce in a large salad bowl. Add the fennel, apple, and scallions. Arrange the green beans on top. Garnish with the grated carrot. When ready to serve, shake the dressing, add it to the salad, and toss well.

Kilocalories 237 Kc • Protein 2 gm • Fat 20 gm • Percent of calories from fat 72% • Cholesterol 0 mg • Dietary fiber 4 gm • Sodium 70 mg • Calcium 60 mg

SALADS

Green Bean and Butternut Salad

―――――――――――――― ■ ――――――――――――――

MAKES 6 SERVINGS

This unusual mixture of flavors is definitely delicious. It's important not to overcook the vegetables.

½ pound fresh green beans, ends trimmed, cut diagonally into 2-inch pieces
¾ pound peeled butternut squash, cut into 2-inch sticks

6 scallions, cut diagonally into 1-inch pieces

For the dressing

3 tablespoons peanut or canola oil
2 tablespoons rice vinegar
1 tablespoon naturally brewed reduced-sodium soy sauce
1 teaspoon sesame oil

½ teaspoon sugar
¼ teaspoon salt
1 slice fresh ginger, very finely minced, or ½ teaspoon ground ginger

Cook the beans in boiling salted water until tender-crisp, 5 to 6 minutes. Remove them with a slotted spoon, saving the water, and rinse them in cold water. Blanch the squash the same way, until just tender, 3 to 5 minutes. Drain and rinse in cold water. When the vegetables are cool, mix them with the scallions in a salad bowl.

Combine all the dressing ingredients in a jar and shake until well blended. Pour the dressing over the vegetables and chill until ready to serve.

Kilocalories 106 Kc • Protein 1 gm • Fat 8 gm • Percent of calories from fat 64% • Cholesterol 0 mg • Dietary fiber 3 gm • Sodium 201 mg • Calcium 30 mg

Chinese Green Bean Salad

This makes a terrific side dish to serve with almost any chicken dish. Try it with Acorn Squash Stuffed with Curried Chicken (page 119).

1 pound fresh green beans, ends trimmed

2 tablespoons sesame seeds

2 tablespoons canola oil

1 teaspoon sesame oil

2 tablespoons rice vinegar

1 teaspoon naturally brewed reduced-sodium soy sauce

1 slice fresh ginger, finely minced, or ¼ teaspoon ground ginger

⅛ teaspoon white pepper

½ teaspoon hot pepper sauce, such as Tabasco (optional)

1 bunch scallions, cut diagonally into 2-inch lengths

4 radishes, thinly sliced

Cook the beans in boiling salted water until tender-crisp, 5 to 6 minutes. Immediately drain and rinse in cold water.

In a small skillet, toast the sesame seeds until they turn golden, about 1 minute, watching them carefully. Remove them from the pan promptly so that the remaining heat will not brown them.

Whisk together the canola oil, sesame oil, rice vinegar, soy sauce, ginger, white pepper, and hot pepper sauce.

In a salad bowl, combine the green beans, scallions, and radishes. Toss with the dressing. Sprinkle with the toasted sesame seeds and serve at once.

Kilocalories 140 Kc • Protein 3 gm • Fat 11 gm • Percent of calories from fat 67% • Cholesterol 0 mg • Dietary fiber 4 gm • Sodium 76 mg • Calcium 84 mg

SALADS

Pinto Bean, Artichoke, and Tomato Salad

■

MAKES 4 SERVINGS

Serve this salad as is or on romaine lettuce leaves. Leftovers make a great pita pocket filler for lunch.

1 (9-ounce) package frozen artichoke hearts

2 cups homemade pinto beans (page 16) or 1 (15- to 16-ounce) can low-sodium pinto beans, drained and rinsed

4 plum tomatoes, seeded and chopped

1 celery stalk with leaves, diced

¼ cup chopped red onion or scallions

2 tablespoons minced fresh flat-leaf parsley

Several fresh basil leaves, chopped, or ½ teaspoon dried

¼ teaspoon salt

Freshly ground black pepper

¼ cup olive oil

3 tablespoons or more red wine vinegar

Romaine lettuce leaves (optional)

Cook the artichoke hearts according to package directions. Drain, rinse, and cool them. Cut into quarters.

In a large salad bowl, mix the artichoke hearts, beans, tomatoes, celery, onion, parsley, basil and salt and pepper to taste. Pour the oil and vinegar over all, and toss well. Taste to see if you want more vinegar. Serve on romaine lettuce leaves, if desired.

Kilocalories 293 Kc • Protein 11 gm • Fat 14 gm • Percent of calories from fat 41% • Cholesterol 0 mg • Dietary fiber 13 gm • Sodium 225 mg • Calcium 85 mg

Cannellini, Bell Pepper, and Tomato Salad

■

MAKES 4 SERVINGS

Fresh crusty Italian bread makes the ideal accompaniment.

1 tablespoon olive oil

1 green bell pepper, seeded and cut into chunks

2 cups homemade cannellini (page 16) or 1 (15- to 16-ounce) can cannellini, drained and rinsed

1 large ripe plum tomato, diced

1 celery stalk with leaves, chopped

4 fresh basil leaves, slivered

3 tablespoons extra-virgin olive oil

2 tablespoons red wine vinegar

¼ teaspoon salt

Freshly ground black pepper

Heat 1 tablespoon oil in a medium skillet and sauté the bell pepper until tender-crisp, 3 to 5 minutes. Cool.

In a large salad bowl, combine the bell pepper, beans, tomato, celery, basil, extra-virgin olive oil, vinegar and salt and pepper to taste. Toss and let stand at room temperature for 20 minutes or so before serving. Taste to correct the seasoning, adding more oil, vinegar, or salt if you wish.

Kilocalories 250 Kc • Protein 9 gm • Fat 14 gm • Percent of calories from fat 49% • Cholesterol 0 mg • Dietary fiber 10 gm • Sodium 165 mg • Calcium 59 mg

Chickpea and Carrot Salad with Whole Wheat Croutons

This is a luncheon salad that goes well with some low-fat cottage cheese or ricotta on the side.

¼ cup olive oil

2 to 3 tablespoons white wine vinegar, to taste

⅛ teaspoon salt

⅛ teaspoon freshly ground black pepper

⅛ teaspoon sugar

1 garlic clove, peeled and halved

1 cup homemade chickpeas (page 16) or canned low-sodium chickpeas, drained and rinsed

1 large carrot, coarsely grated

4 scallions, chopped

1 small to medium head red leaf lettuce

1 cup Whole Wheat Croutons (page 311)

In a jar, combine the oil, vinegar, salt, pepper, sugar, and garlic. Cover and shake to blend the dressing. Allow it to marinate for a half hour or more. Shake again just before using.

Pour the dressing through a small strainer into the bottom of a salad bowl; discard the garlic. Stir the chickpeas, carrot, and scallions into the dressing. Put the lettuce on top, but don't toss the salad. Chill until ready to serve. Toss the salad just before serving and sprinkle with the croutons.

Kilocalories 243 Kc • Protein 5 gm • Fat 17 gm • Percent of calories from fat 60% • Cholesterol 0 mg • Dietary fiber 5 gm • Sodium 125 mg • Calcium 75 mg

Whole Wheat Croutons

These are so much less fatty and salty than the store-bought ones!

2 slices firm whole wheat bread   **1 garlic clove, sliced in half**
1 tablespoon olive oil
1 teaspoon Italian seasoning or a
  mixture of dried basil,
  oregano, rosemary, and thyme

Preheat the oven to 250 degrees F.

Trim off the crusts and dice the bread. Toss the bread cubes with the oil and herbs. Make one layer of cubes in a baking pan, add the garlic, and bake, stirring once or twice, until the croutons are crispy but not over-browned, about 20 minutes. Discard the garlic and cool the croutons. Store them in a covered jar for up to a week.

Kilocalories 33 Kc • Protein 1 gm • Fat 2 gm • Percent of calories from fat 52% • Cholesterol 0 mg • Dietary fiber 1 gm • Sodium 37 mg • Calcium 9 mg

SALADS

Lentil, Tomato, and Scallion Salad

■

MAKES 4 SERVINGS

Try this as a make-ahead buffet salad.

1 cup lentils, picked over and
  rinsed
1 garlic clove, halved
½ teaspoon salt
2 medium tomatoes, diced small
4 scallions, chopped
1 celery stalk with leaves,
  chopped

3 tablespoons extra-virgin
  olive oil
2 tablespoons red wine vinegar
Freshly ground black pepper
1 tablespoon minced fresh flat-
  leaf parsley
1 teaspoon chopped fresh mint

Combine the lentils, 3 cups of water, garlic, and salt in a saucepan. Bring to a boil and simmer, uncovered, until the lentils are just tender but still retain their shape, 25 to 30 minutes. Drain and rinse in cool water. Remove and discard the garlic.

In a salad bowl, mix the lentils, tomatoes, scallions, and celery. Add the oil and vinegar with pepper to taste. Stir in the parsley and mint. Let the salad stand at room temperature for 15 to 20 minutes before serving.

Kilocalories 270 Kc • Protein 14 gm • Fat 11 gm • Percent of calories from fat 35% • Cholesterol 0 mg • Dietary fiber 16 gm • Sodium 317 mg • Calcium 43 mg

Navy Bean Salad with Scallions

■

MAKES 4 SERVINGS

When homemade beans are not available, cooked frozen beans, a new product on the market, are a wonderful quick way to make a fresh-tasting bean salad.

2 cups homemade navy beans
    (page 16) or 1 (14-ounce)
    package frozen navy beans,
    thawed
½ cup finely diced red bell
    pepper

4 scallions, finely chopped
1 tablespoon chopped fresh flat-
    leaf parsley
⅓ cup Garlic and Lemon
    Vinaigrette (page 19)

Combine all the ingredients and let stand at room temperature for 20 minutes to blend the flavors.

Kilocalories 291 Kc • Protein 9 gm • Fat 18 gm • Percent of calories from fat
54% • Cholesterol 0 mg • Dietary fiber 10 gm • Sodium 55 mg • Calcium 68 mg

Beet Salad with Mint

■

MAKES 4 SERVINGS

Serve chilled or at room temperature as you wish—it's good either way.

2 bunches beets (6 to 8), well
    scrubbed (reserve the greens
    for another use)
½ cup chopped sweet onion,
    such as Vidalia, or chopped
    scallions

2 tablespoons minced fresh mint
¼ teaspoon salt
Freshly ground black pepper
3 tablespoons olive oil
2 tablespoons fresh lemon juice

Put the beets in a saucepan with water to cover and boil them until tender,
about 30 minutes. Remove them with a slotted spoon. When they are cool
enough to handle, peel and slice them. Put the slices in a shallow dish.

    Add the onion, mint and salt and pepper to taste. Drizzle the salad with
the oil and lemon juice, and toss the salad very, very gently. Let the salad
marinate for a half hour or more.

Kilocalories 208 Kc • Protein 4 gm • Fat 11 gm • Percent of calories from fat
43% • Cholesterol 0 mg • Dietary fiber 8 gm • Sodium 323 mg • Calcium 49 mg

Beet Salad with Balsamic Vinegar

■

MAKES 4 SERVINGS, WITH SOME LEFTOVER BEETS

The attractive color contrast in this salad makes it a nice show-off "company for dinner" salad.

About 4 large beets, well
  scrubbed (reserve the greens
  for another use)
1 teaspoon salt
1 sweet onion, such as Vidalia,
  chopped
¼ teaspoon freshly ground black
  pepper

½ cup balsamic vinegar
4 cups bite-size chicory or
  romaine lettuce pieces
About 4 tablespoons extra-virgin
  olive oil

Put the beets in a large saucepan with the salt and water to cover, bring to a simmer, and cook, covered, until the beets are tender, about 45 minutes. Cool the beets. Strain the liquid through a paper coffee filter set into a strainer over a bowl.

Peel the beets, cut them in half, then slice into half rounds. Put them in a deep bowl with the onion and pepper. Add enough of the liquid to nearly reach the top of the slices. Add the vinegar and stir gently. Chill the beets.

Divide the salad greens among 4 plates. Top each with about ¾ cup of the beets and 2 tablespoons of the juice. Drizzle oil over each serving.

Kilocalories 297 Kc • Protein 6 gm • Fat 14 gm • Percent of calories from fat 42% • Cholesterol 0 mg • Dietary fiber 14 gm • Sodium 802 mg • Calcium 222 mg

ANTIOXIDANT POWER

Broccoli de Rabe Salad with Lemon Vinaigrette

MAKES 4 SERVINGS

Cooked greens served as a salad is characteristic of North African cookery.

1 bunch broccoli de rabe,
  washed, tough stems removed,
  chopped into thirds (¾ pound)
3 tablespoons olive oil
2 tablespoons fresh lemon juice
1 tablespoon chopped fresh
  marjoram or ½ teaspoon dried
  oregano

¼ teaspoon salt
⅛ teaspoon freshly ground black
  pepper
1 large carrot, shredded

Combine the broccoli de rabe and ½ cup water in a pot, bring to a simmer, and cook, covered, until the broccoli de rabe is tender, 10 to 15 minutes. Drain and spoon the broccoli de rabe into a serving dish and allow it to cool.

Whisk together the oil, lemon juice, marjoram or oregano, salt, and pepper, and pour the dressing over the broccoli de rabe. Top with the shredded carrot. Serve at room temperature.

Kilocalories 137 Kc • Protein 3 gm • Fat 10 gm • Percent of calories from fat 66% • Cholesterol 0 mg • Dietary fiber 1 gm • Sodium 169 mg • Calcium 163 mg

Hot Cabbage Salad

Seeds can be crushed with a pestle in a mortar, with the back of a heavy frying pan, or with an old-fashioned wooden mallet for mashing potatoes, one of my favorite kitchen tools, which is also useful for smashing garlic for easy peeling.

2 (¼-inch) slices pancetta
  (Italian bacon), finely diced
1 teaspoon olive oil
1 medium yellow onion, sliced
  and separated into rings
6 cups finely shredded cabbage,
  loosely packed
1 teaspoon fennel seeds,
  crushed

¼ cup broth or water
2 tablespoons or more white
  wine vinegar
¼ teaspoon salt (optional)
¼ teaspoon freshly ground black
  pepper

In a nonstick unoiled 12-inch skillet, cook the pancetta over medium heat until it's crisp and brown, 3 to 5 minutes. Remove the pancetta and drain it between paper towels. Discard the fat and clean out the pan. Add the oil and sauté the onion until it's soft and lightly colored, 3 to 5 minutes.

Add the cabbage, fennel seeds, and broth or water. Cook, uncovered, over medium heat, stirring constantly, until the cabbage has just wilted to half its original size, about 3 minutes. Immediately remove from the heat. Stir in the pancetta and vinegar. Add salt, if using, and pepper. Taste to see if you want more vinegar. Serve hot or at room temperature.

Kilocalories 118 Kc • Protein 6 gm • Fat 7 gm • Percent of calories from fat 49% • Cholesterol 10 mg • Dietary fiber 3 gm • Sodium 272 mg • Calcium 68 mg

ANTIOXIDANT POWER

316

Picnic Coleslaw

Not your pale, mayonnaise-drenched, sugary deli slaw, this one is full of colorful, antioxidant-rich carrots, plus the abundant vitamin C in the cabbage. A good coleslaw depends on the thinness of the cabbage, so if you have a shredder appliance, use it for this salad.

¼ cup mayonnaise
¼ cup nonfat plain yogurt
1 tablespoon minced fresh dill
   or ½ teaspoon dried
¼ teaspoon celery salt
¼ teaspoon white pepper

½ pound cabbage, very thinly
   shredded (½ head)
2 large carrots, coarsely grated
¼ cup chopped sweet or
   red onion

Whisk together the mayonnaise, yogurt, dill, celery salt, and pepper. Toss with the cabbage, carrots, and onion. Chill for several hours to develop the flavor. Toss again before serving.

Kilocalories 95 Kc • Protein 1 gm • Fat 8 gm • Percent of calories from fat 69% • Cholesterol 7 mg • Dietary fiber 2 gm • Sodium 73 mg • Calcium 46 mg

Pineapple Coleslaw

This is a great favorite with kids. They hardly realize what wonderful vegetables they're enjoying.

¼ cup canola oil
2 tablespoons rice vinegar
½ teaspoon salt
⅛ teaspoon white pepper
½ pound cabbage, very thinly
  shredded (½ head)

2 carrots, coarsely grated
1 (8-ounce) can juice-packed
  crushed pineapple, undrained
¼ cup golden raisins

Whisk together the oil, vinegar, salt, and pepper. Toss with the cabbage, carrots, pineapple, and raisins. Chill for several hours to develop the flavor. Toss again before serving.

Kilocalories 147 Kc • Protein 1 gm • Fat 10 gm • Percent of calories from fat 56% • Cholesterol 0 mg • Dietary fiber 2 gm • Sodium 211 mg • Calcium 40 mg

Caesar's Coleslaw

This coleslaw has a definitely grown-up flavor for those who love the tang of anchovies.

½ pound cabbage, very thinly
  shredded (½ head)
2 large carrots, coarsely grated
¼ cup chopped sweet or
  red onion

½ cup Caesar Salad Dressing
  with Roasted Garlic (page 21),
  or more, to taste.

Put all the ingredients in a mixing bowl and toss well. Transfer the salad to a serving dish and chill until needed.

Kilocalories 152 Kc • Protein 2 gm • Fat 14 gm • Percent of calories from fat 80% • Cholesterol 1 mg • Dietary fiber 2 gm • Sodium 65 mg • Calcium 36 mg

Carrot Slaw with Scallions

---◼---

MAKES 6 SERVINGS

This slaw is an attractive combination of vivid colors.

1 pound carrots, coarsely grated
1 bunch scallions with green
   tops, chopped
2 tablespoons finely minced
   fresh flat-leaf parsley

½ cup Dijon Vinaigrette
   (page 20)
About 6 outer red cabbage
   leaves

Toss together the carrots, scallions, and parsley. Pour the dressing over the vegetables and toss to coat evenly. Chill. When ready to serve, arrange the red cabbage leaves in a salad dish and heap the carrot slaw in the center.

Kilocalories 156 Kc • Protein 2 gm • Fat 11 gm • Percent of calories from fat 58% • Cholesterol 0 mg • Dietary fiber 4 gm • Sodium 61 mg • Calcium 63 mg

Carrot Slaw with Pineapple and Raisins

MAKES **6** SERVINGS

Serve this as a kid-pleasing antioxidant-packed side dish or tuck it into a whole wheat pita pocket for a snack.

2 pounds carrots, coarsely grated
1 (8-ounce) can juice-packed crushed pineapple, undrained

3 tablespoons vegetable oil
¼ teaspoon salt
¼ cup raisins

Toss together the carrots, pineapple, oil, and salt to blend evenly. Stir in the raisins. Chill.

Kilocalories 134 Kc • Protein 1 gm • Fat 7 gm • Percent of calories from fat 45% • Cholesterol 0 mg • Dietary fiber 3 gm • Sodium 124 mg • Calcium 29 mg

Carrot and Bell Pepper Salad

This sweet-and-sour favorite would team well with braised or roasted chicken.

1 pound carrots, cut diagonally
   into 1-inch pieces
2 tablespoons olive oil
2 green bell peppers, seeded
   and diced
⅓ cup cider vinegar

⅓ cup sugar
¼ teaspoon salt
⅓ cup chili sauce
½ teaspoon dry mustard
½ cup chopped red onion

Cook the carrots in boiling salted water until tender, about 5 minutes. Drain and rinse in cool water.

Heat the oil in a medium skillet and stir-fry the bell peppers until tender-crisp, 3 to 5 minutes.

In a small saucepan, warm the vinegar and stir in the sugar and salt until they are dissolved. Blend in the chili sauce and mustard.

Combine the carrots, bell peppers, and red onion in a large salad bowl. Toss with the vinegar mixture. Chill for an hour or more before serving.

Kilocalories 145 Kc • Protein 2 gm • Fat 5 gm • Percent of calories from fat 29% • Cholesterol 0 mg • Dietary fiber 3 gm • Sodium 133 mg • Calcium 31 mg

Southwestern Corn, Bean, and Cabbage Salad

_____◼_____

MAKES 6 SERVINGS, OR MORE AS PART OF A BUFFET

A savory chopped salad like this is a popular choice for picnics and buffets.

2 cups finely chopped romaine lettuce

2 cups fresh cooked corn, cut from the cob

1 cup homemade black beans (page 16) or canned low-sodium black beans, drained and rinsed

1 cup finely chopped red cabbage

½ cup finely chopped sweet onion

1 or 2 fresh or canned jalapeño chilies, seeded and minced (wear rubber gloves)

2 tablespoons chopped fresh cilantro

1 tablespoon pepitas (shelled pumpkin seeds, available in natural food stores—optional)

3 tablespoons canola oil

2 tablespoons lime juice

½ teaspoon salt

Several grindings of black pepper

Baked tortilla chips for garnish (optional)

In a large bowl, toss together all the ingredients except the chips. Chill to blend the flavors. Taste to correct the seasoning. You may want more canola oil, lime juice, or salt. Serve with chips on the side.

Kilocalories 163 Kc • Protein 5 gm • Fat 8 gm • Percent of calories from fat 43% • Cholesterol 0 mg • Dietary fiber 4 gm • Sodium 229 mg • Calcium 37 mg

Herbed Baby Carrot Salad

———— ◼ ————

Cooked vegetable salads are great make-aheads for quick supper side dishes.

1 (1-pound) bag peeled baby
  carrots
½ cup nonfat plain yogurt
2 tablespoons mayonnaise
¼ teaspoon celery salt

¼ teaspoon white pepper
3 tablespoons chopped fresh
  chives or fresh dill or a
  combination

Put the carrots in a saucepan with water to cover and boil until they are tender, about 15 minutes. Drain well and cool.

Whisk together all the remaining ingredients. Stir in the carrots. Chill to blend the flavors.

Kilocalories 74 Kc • Protein 2 gm • Fat 4 gm • Percent of calories from fat 49% • Cholesterol 3 mg • Dietary fiber 1 gm • Sodium 66 mg • Calcium 57 mg

Key West Carrots

6 large carrots, cut in julienne
1 celery stalk, cut in julienne
2 tablespoons vegetable oil
Juice of 1 large lime (2 to
  3 tablespoons)

¼ teaspoon salt
⅛ teaspoon white pepper
1 garlic clove, very finely minced
Lime wedges for garnish

Blanch the carrots in a large pot of boiling salted water for 1 minute. Drain and rinse in cold water until the carrots are cool to the touch. Combine the carrots and celery in a salad bowl.

Whisk together the oil, lime juice, salt, pepper, and garlic. Toss the salad with the dressing. Let stand at room temperature for 15 minutes before serving. Garnish with the lime wedges.

Kilocalories 74 Kc • Protein 1 gm • Fat 5 gm • Percent of calories from fat 54% • Cholesterol 0 mg • Dietary fiber 2 gm • Sodium 128 mg • Calcium 24 mg

Cauliflower and Tomato Salad

Always shake a vinaigrette just before measuring to mix the vinegar and oil.

1 medium head cauliflower,
  separated into florets (cut
  extra large florets in half)
1 pint cherry tomatoes, halved
6 scallions with green tops,
  chopped

1 (4-ounce) can pitted black
  olives, drained
¼ to ⅓ cup Garlic and Lemon
  Vinaigrette (page 19)

ANTIOXIDANT POWER

324

Cook the cauliflower in boiling salted water until tender-crisp, about 3 minutes. Drain and rinse in cold water until cool to the touch.

Toss together the cauliflower, tomatoes, scallions, olives, and dressing. Start with ¼ cup of dressing and taste to see if you want more.

Kilocalories 138 Kc • Protein 4 gm • Fat 11 gm • Percent of calories from fat 65% • Cholesterol 0 mg • Dietary fiber 5 gm • Sodium 250 mg • Calcium 58 mg

Fennel and Bell Pepper Salad

———————————■———————————

MAKES 6 SERVINGS

As soon as the fennel is chopped, mix it with the vinaigrette to prevent browning.

½ cup or more Herb Vinaigrette (page 20)
2 large fennel bulbs, cored and chopped, leaves reserved for garnish (2 pounds)

1 green bell pepper, seeded and diced
12 cherry tomatoes, halved
¼ cup finely chopped red onion
Romaine lettuce leaves

Pour the vinaigrette into a salad bowl. Stir in the fennel. Toss with the green peppers, tomatoes, and onions. Chill until ready to serve. Toss again and add more vinaigrette if desired.

To serve, mound the salad on lettuce leaves and garnish with fennel leaves.

Kilocalories 133 Kc • Protein 1 gm • Fat 12 gm • Percent of calories from fat 80% • Cholesterol 0 mg • Dietary fiber 2 gm • Sodium 116 mg • Calcium 23 mg

Apple and Fennel Salad

■

MAKES 6 SERVINGS

This is possibly the perfect salad to accompany a roast loin of pork.

¼ cup canola oil

2 to 3 tablespoons cider vinegar, to taste

½ teaspoon sugar

¼ teaspoon salt

⅛ teaspoon white pepper

2 medium unpeeled red-skinned apples, such as Rome, Gala, McIntosh, or Macoun

1 small fennel bulb, trimmed and cored, plus about ½ cup chopped fennel leaves, called "hair"

6 cups bite-size mixed greens (choose 2 from: romaine, red leaf lettuce, chicory, baby spinach)

In the bottom of a large salad bowl, whisk together the oil, vinegar, sugar, salt, and pepper. Core the apples and dice them into the vinaigrette; this will prevent them from turning brown. Do the same with the fennel bulb. Gently toss to coat all sides with the vinaigrette.

Add the greens and fennel hair to the bowl without tossing; this will keep it crisp until serving time. Chill the salad until ready to serve. Taste to see if you want more oil or vinegar.

Kilocalories 124 Kc • Protein 2 gm • Fat 10 gm • Percent of calories from fat 65% • Cholesterol 0 mg • Dietary fiber 3 gm • Sodium 130 mg • Calcium 63 mg

Potato and Spinach Salad with Yogurt Dressing

■

A boiling potato has a thin red or tan skin and a round shape; it's also known as a waxy potato. It tends to hold its shape through cooking, making it a good choice for potato salad.

½ cup nonfat plain yogurt
¼ cup mayonnaise
2 tablespoons chopped fresh dill
  or 1 teaspoon dried
¼ teaspoon celery salt
¼ teaspoon white pepper
1 pound fresh spinach, washed,
  tough stems removed

4 large boiling potatoes, peeled
  and cut into 1-inch cubes
  (about 1½ pounds)
2 garlic cloves, peeled
2 celery stalks with leaves, diced
Fresh dill sprigs for garnish
  (optional)

In a small deep bowl, whisk together the yogurt, mayonnaise, dill, celery salt, and white pepper until smooth.

In a large pot, wilt the spinach in just the water that clings to the leaves after washing; drain.

Steam the potatoes with the garlic until tender, about 10 minutes; drain. Mash the garlic very well and incorporate it evenly into the dressing.

In a large bowl, toss the potatoes and celery with the dressing. Layer the spinach on a platter. Spread the potato mixture on top. Garnish with dill sprigs, if desired. Serve at room temperature or chilled.

Kilocalories 197 Kc • Protein 6 gm • Fat 8 gm • Percent of calories from fat 34% • Cholesterol 7 mg • Dietary fiber 4 gm • Sodium 140 mg • Calcium 126 mg

SALADS

Potato and Dandelion Salad

Vinegar in the water keeps boiling potatoes from turning dark.

4 large boiling potatoes, peeled
   and cut into 1-inch cubes
   (about 1½ pounds)
1 tablespoon white vinegar
¼ cup finely chopped red or
   white sweet onion
2 inner celery stalks with leaves,
   chopped

3 tablespoons red wine vinegar
4 tablespoons extra-virgin
   olive oil
¼ teaspoon salt
Freshly ground black pepper
2 cups well-washed chopped
   dandelion greens (about
   ⅓ pound)

Put the potatoes in a saucepan with water to cover. Add the white vinegar. Bring to a boil, reduce the heat, and simmer, covered, until tender, 5 to 7 minutes. Drain well and cool.

In a salad bowl, combine the potatoes, onion, and celery. Add 2 tablespoons of the wine vinegar and toss well. Add 3 tablespoons of the oil, salt, and pepper to taste, and toss again. Put the dandelion greens on top (don't mix yet) and chill the salad.

When ready to serve, add the remaining tablespoon of vinegar and tablespoon of oil. Toss, blending in the greens. Taste to correct the seasoning. You may want more oil, vinegar, or salt.

Kilocalories 195 Kc • Protein 3 gm • Fat 9 gm • Percent of calories from fat 42% • Cholesterol 0 mg • Dietary fiber 3 gm • Sodium 129 mg • Calcium 64 mg

ANTIOXIDANT POWER

Red Potato and Watercress Salad

Potato skins are richer in vitamins than any other part of the potato. When using unpeeled potatoes, carefully remove any blemishes that don't scrub off and cut out any sprouts.

4 large unpeeled red potatoes, well scrubbed and cut into 1-inch pieces (about 1½ pounds)
1 tablespoon white vinegar
1 tablespoon olive oil
1 red bell pepper, seeded and cut into 1-inch chunks
½ cup finely chopped red onion

¼ cup mayonnaise
½ cup nonfat plain yogurt
2 teaspoons Dijon mustard
1 tablespoon chopped fresh dill or ½ teaspoon dried
¼ teaspoon celery salt
¼ teaspoon white pepper
1 bunch watercress, tougher stems removed, chopped

Put the potatoes in a saucepan with water to cover. Add the white vinegar. Bring to a boil, reduce the heat, and simmer, covered, until tender, 5 to 7 minutes. Drain well and cool.

In a small skillet, heat the oil and fry the pepper, stirring often, until tender-crisp, 3 to 5 minutes. In a large bowl, mix the potatoes, red bell pepper, and onion.

Whisk together the mayonnaise, yogurt, mustard, dill, celery salt, and white pepper. Stir about two thirds of the dressing into the vegetables. Chill until ready to serve (at least 1 hour). When ready to serve, stir in the remaining dressing and the watercress.

Kilocalories 210 Kc • Protein 4 gm • Fat 10 gm • Percent of calories from fat 41% • Cholesterol 7 mg • Dietary fiber 3 gm • Sodium 93 mg • Calcium 90 mg

Potato and Broccoli Salad with Dijon Dressing

MAKES 6 SERVINGS

Zesty Dijon mustard stands up to the strong flavor of broccoli and makes a delicious salad that combines two of the great cancer-fighting vegetables.

2 tablespoons Dijon mustard
2 tablespoons white wine vinegar
¼ teaspoon white pepper
About ½ cup vegetable oil (can be olive oil or a blend)
4 large boiling potatoes, peeled and cut into 1-inch cubes (about 1½ pounds)

1 tablespoon white vinegar
1 pound fresh broccoli, cut into florets and ½-inch slices of stalk
1 celery stalk with leaves, diced
4 to 6 scallions with green tops, chopped
2 tablespoons chopped fresh dill or 1 teaspoon dried

Combine the mustard, wine vinegar, and pepper in a small deep bowl. Gradually whisk the oil into the mustard mixture until the dressing is smooth and emulsified. Alternatively, a stationary or hand blender can be used to make this step easier.

Put the potatoes in a saucepan with water to cover. Add the white vinegar. Bring to a boil, reduce the heat, and simmer, covered, until tender, 5 to 7 minutes. Drain well and cool.

Cook the broccoli in boiling salted water until tender-crisp, 2 to 3 minutes. Drain and rinse in cold water.

Combine the potatoes, broccoli, celery, scallions, and dill in a salad bowl, and toss with the dressing. Chill until needed.

Kilocalories 291 Kc • Protein 5 gm • Fat 19 gm • Percent of calories from fat 56% • Cholesterol 0 mg • Dietary fiber 5 gm • Sodium 61 mg • Calcium 58 mg

ANTIOXIDANT POWER

Sweet Potato and Pancetta Salad

This unusual potato salad has a distinctively Mediterranean flavor.

2 (¼-inch) slices pancetta
2 large sweet potatoes, peeled
  and quartered lengthwise
  (about 1½ pounds)
4 shallots or 2 large garlic
  cloves, peeled and halved
3 tablespoons canola oil

2 tablespoons cider vinegar
1 teaspoon chopped fresh thyme
  or ¼ teaspoon dried
⅛ teaspoon salt
⅛ teaspoon freshly ground black
  pepper

In a nonstick unoiled 10-inch skillet, cook the pancetta over medium heat until it's crisp and brown, 3 to 5 minutes. Remove the pancetta and drain it between paper towels. Discard the fat.

Steam the potatoes with the shallots until tender, 10 to 15 minutes; drain. Cool slightly. Slice the potatoes into half rounds. Chop the shallots.

Whisk together the oil, vinegar, thyme, salt, and pepper. Gently toss the potatoes, shallots, and pancetta with the dressing. (If you substitute garlic, be sure to distribute it evenly throughout.) Serve at room temperature.

Kilocalories 299 Kc • Protein 7 gm • Fat 16 gm • Percent of calories from fat 46% • Cholesterol 10 mg • Dietary fiber 3 gm • Sodium 330 mg • Calcium 23 mg

Butternut, Red Cabbage, and Blue Cheese Salad

MAKES 4 SERVINGS

For the adventurous cook—this unusual combination is a powerhouse of antioxidants, and very colorful, as well!

**2 cups 1-inch butternut
  squash cubes
2 cups shredded red cabbage
4 scallions, chopped**

**⅓ cup crumbled blue cheese
About ½ cup Herb Vinaigrette
  (page 20)**

Steam the squash until it's just tender, about 8 minutes. Cool completely.

In a salad bowl, combine the squash, red cabbage, scallions, and blue cheese. Toss with ½ cup of the dressing and allow the salad to marinate at room temperature for 20 minutes or so before serving. Taste to determine if you want more vinaigrette.

Kilocalories 170 Kc • Protein 4 gm • Fat 15 gm • Percent of calories from fat 74% • Cholesterol 7 mg • Dietary fiber 2 gm • Sodium 236 mg • Calcium 86 mg

Individual Tomato Salads, Italian Style

Called panzanella *(bread salad), this quick summer dish includes fresh "croutons" to sop up the flavorful juices.*

4 large juicy vine-ripened
tomatoes, cut into wedges
(2 pounds total)
1 cup chopped Vidalia onion
8 large fresh basil leaves,
snipped
Salt and freshly ground black
pepper

About 4 tablespoons extra-virgin
olive oil
2 large thick slices Italian bread
with crusts, diced
4 fresh basil sprigs for garnish
(optional)

In 4 individual salad bowls, arrange the tomatoes and sprinkle them with the chopped onion and basil. Season with salt and pepper to taste. (Salt draws juice out of the tomatoes.) Drizzle on the olive oil, stir, and allow the salads to marinate for 20 minutes. Divide the bread among the dishes and stir. Garnish with basil sprigs, if desired.

Kilocalories 201 Kc • Protein 3 gm • Fat 15 gm • Percent of calories from fat 63% • Cholesterol 0 mg • Dietary fiber 3 gm • Sodium 100 mg • Calcium 27 mg

SALADS

Tomato and Roasted Bell Pepper Salad

MAKES 4 SERVINGS

Although substitution is possible, the delectable flavor of homemade roasted peppers cannot be equaled by their store-bought counterparts.

2 large green bell peppers
3 tablespoons extra-virgin
  olive oil
1 garlic clove, halved
1 tablespoon chopped fresh
  basil or 1 teaspoon dried

1 teaspoon chopped fresh mint
¼ teaspoon salt
4 ripe tomatoes, cut into wedges

A few hours before making the salad, prepare and marinate the peppers. Preheat the broiler. Broil the peppers 6 inches below the heat source, turning often, until they are tender when pressed and somewhat charred on all sides, 2 to 3 minutes per side. Put the peppers into a covered dish. When they are cool enough to handle, peel off the skins, seed them, and cut them into strips. Return them to the dish and add the oil, garlic, herbs, and salt. Allow the peppers to marinate at room temperature about 45 minutes.

Remove the garlic, add the tomatoes, and toss. Continue to let stand about 15 minutes before serving.

Kilocalories 127 Kc • Protein 1 gm • Fat 11 gm • Percent of calories from fat 71% • Cholesterol 0 mg • Dietary fiber 2 gm • Sodium 157 mg • Calcium 13 mg

"Deep Summer" Tomato Salad with Scallions

This salad is so simple and so delicious. Everything depends on having local farm-grown, vine-ripened tomatoes—it's even better if you grow your own! The juice drawn out of the tomatoes by salting them combines with the oil to make a vinaigrette.

**4 perfectly ripe beefsteak
   tomatoes, sliced**
**4 scallions with green tops,
   chopped**
Salt

**3 tablespoons extra-virgin
   olive oil**
**Fresh white Italian bread as an
   accompaniment**

In a flat dish with a lip, combine the tomato slices and scallions. Salt them to taste and drizzle with olive oil. Let stand for a half hour, using 2 forks to carefully turn the tomatoes and scallions in the oil once. Serve with fresh bread on the side.

Kilocalories 117 Kc • Protein 1 gm • Fat 11 gm • Percent of calories from fat 76% • Cholesterol 0 mg • Dietary fiber 2 gm • Sodium 12 mg • Calcium 10 mg

Tomato, Fennel, and Olive Salad

MAKES 4 SERVINGS

Here's an antipasto-style salad you can make in the fall when the only good tomatoes are plum tomatoes but lots of nice fresh fennel has come into the market.

2 cups seeded chopped ripe plum tomatoes
½ cup pitted chopped green Sicilian olives
3 tablespoons extra-virgin olive oil

1 garlic clove, very finely minced
Freshly ground black pepper
1 large fennel bulb, quartered, cored, and diced, plus a few feathery sprays of chopped fennel leaves

In a salad bowl, combine the tomatoes, olives, oil, and garlic, stirring carefully to distribute the garlic evenly. Add pepper to taste; the olives provide the salt.

Stir in the diced fennel. Allow the salad to marinate at room temperature for a half hour before serving. Sprinkle with the chopped fennel leaves.

Kilocalories 138 Kc • Protein 1 gm • Fat 12 gm • Percent of calories from fat 75% • Cholesterol 0 mg • Dietary fiber 2 gm • Sodium 310 mg • Calcium 24 mg

Sautéed Squash and Bell Pepper Salad

This ample salad might be a lunchtime entrée, accompanied by a wedge of assertive cheese, such as aged provolone, and a fresh crusty loaf of bread.

2 tablespoons olive oil
1 pound summer and zucchini
  squash, sliced diagonally
  (about 3 small mixed squash)
1 red bell pepper, seeded and
  cut into 2-inch sticks
2 large shallots, chopped
¼ teaspoon dried oregano

¼ teaspoon salt
Freshly ground black pepper
2 tablespoons balsamic vinegar
4 to 6 cups salad greens, torn
  into bite-size pieces (romaine
  and chicory, for instance)
About 4 teaspoons extra-virgin
  olive oil

Heat the oil in a 12-inch skillet, and stir-fry the squash and bell pepper until lightly browned and tender-crisp, 5 to 8 minutes. Add the shallots during the last 3 minutes. Season with oregano, salt, and pepper to taste. Sprinkle with the vinegar.

Divide the greens among 4 large salad plates. Top with the squash. Drizzle on extra-virgin olive oil to taste.

Kilocalories 156 Kc • Protein 3 gm • Fat 12 gm • Percent of calories from fat 64% • Cholesterol 0 mg • Dietary fiber 6 gm • Sodium 193 mg • Calcium 122 mg

SALADS

Braised Vegetable Salad with Lemon-Tarragon Dressing

MAKES 4 SERVINGS

Braised vegetables should be just a little browned on some sides, which gives them a deliciously different flavor.

½ pound carrots, sliced diagonally into 1-inch pieces

2 tablespoons olive oil

2 small zucchini, quartered lengthwise and cut into 1-inch chunks (about 1¼ pounds)

2 celery stalks, sliced diagonally into 1-inch pieces

Salt and freshly ground black pepper

1 teaspoon minced fresh tarragon or ¼ teaspoon dried

2 tablespoons lemon juice (½ lemon)

2 scallions, sliced diagonally into ½-inch pieces (optional)

Nonfat plain yogurt

Parboil the carrots in salted water for 5 minutes. Drain.

Heat 1 tablespoon oil in a nonstick skillet, and braise the carrots, zucchini, and celery until tender-crisp, 5 to 7 minutes. Season to taste with salt and pepper. Stir in the tarragon. Chill the vegetables.

When ready to serve, toss the vegetables with the lemon juice, remaining tablespoon of oil, and the scallions, if using. Serve with yogurt as a topping.

Kilocalories 109 Kc • Protein 2 gm • Fat 7 gm • Percent of calories from fat 54% • Cholesterol 0 mg • Dietary fiber 4 gm • Sodium 42 mg • Calcium 46 mg

Curried Vegetable Salad

■

Here's a savory luncheon entrée. Cheese 'n Wheat Rolls (page 268) or bakery-fresh wheat rolls would be a pleasing accompaniment.

½ head cauliflower, separated into florets

½ pound fresh green beans, ends trimmed, cut diagonally into 2-inch pieces

2 carrots, cut diagonally into 1-inch pieces

2 purple-topped turnips, pared and cut into thin wedges

4 scallions, chopped

For the dressing

¼ cup nonfat plain yogurt

2 tablespoons mayonnaise

1 teaspoon curry powder

¼ teaspoon salt

¼ teaspoon white pepper

Cook the cauliflower, green beans, carrots, and turnips separately in boiling salted water until each is tender-crisp. (Use the same pot of water.) Timing will be about 3 minutes for cauliflower, 5 minutes for green beans, 8 minutes for carrots, and 3 minutes for turnips. They should still be crunchy. Remove with a slotted spoon and rinse in cold water. In a salad bowl, mix the cooled vegetables with the scallions.

Blend the dressing ingredients together and toss the vegetables with the dressing. Chill until ready to serve.

Kilocalories 84 Kc • Protein 3 gm • Fat 4 gm • Percent of calories from fat 40% • Cholesterol 3 mg • Dietary fiber 5 gm • Sodium 182 mg • Calcium 71 mg

Marinated Vegetable Salad

■

MAKES 6 SERVINGS

In this recipe, fresh vegetable "pickles" are served as a topping for greens, but they are also very tasty without greens as a part of an appetizer buffet.

2 cups cauliflower florets, cut small
5 tablespoons cider vinegar
1 tablespoon sugar
½ teaspoon celery salt
3 tablespoons olive oil
½ teaspoon freshly ground black pepper
2 carrots, very thinly sliced

6 to 8 radishes, thinly sliced (1 bunch)
2 celery stalks, thinly sliced
1 cucumber, thinly sliced
1 red onion, thinly sliced and separated into rings
4 cups mixed salad greens, such as romaine, chicory, and/or red leaf lettuce

Parboil the cauliflower in boiling salted water for 1 minute, timing from when the water comes to a second boil after adding the vegetable. Drain and rinse in cold water.

In a small saucepan, combine the vinegar, sugar, and celery salt. Warm the mixture, stirring, just enough to dissolve the sugar and salt. Remove and cool. Stir in the oil and pepper. Pour the dressing into a deep bowl. Add the carrots, cauliflower, radishes, celery, cucumber, and onion. Allow them to marinate at room temperature for a half hour or so, stirring from time to time so that all the vegetables are coated. Chill the vegetables.

Line a large salad bowl with the greens. Heap the vegetables in the center and serve.

Kilocalories 121 Kc • Protein 3 gm • Fat 7 gm • Percent of calories from fat 50% • Cholesterol 0 mg • Dietary fiber 5 gm • Sodium 45 mg • Calcium 76 mg

Orzo Pilaf Salad with Vegetables

■

2 tablespoons olive oil
1 small onion, chopped
½ cup orzo
1 cup long-grain rice
3 cups chicken stock (page 10)
  or canned low-sodium broth
1 cup cooked fresh or
  frozen peas
1 cup seeded diced plum
  tomatoes

4 scallions, finely chopped
1 celery stalk with leaves, finely
  chopped
2 tablespoons minced fresh flat-
  leaf parsley
½ cup Garlic and Lemon
  Vinaigrette (page 19)

Heat the oil in a large heavy saucepan and sauté the onion for 1 minute. Add the orzo and sauté, stirring, until it's lightly colored, ½ minute. Add the rice and stir to coat all the grains with the oil. Add the stock, bring to a simmer, and cook, covered, until the liquid is absorbed, about 18 minutes. Fluff with a fork, spread out on a platter, and cool the pilaf to room temperature.

In a salad bowl, combine the pilaf, peas, tomatoes, scallions, celery, and parsley. Dress the salad with the vinaigrette and toss well. Serve at room temperature.

Kilocalories 612 Kc • Protein 11 gm • Fat 35 gm • Percent of calories from fat 52% • Cholesterol 1 mg • Dietary fiber 5 gm • Sodium 125 mg • Calcium 50 mg

SALADS

Asian Noodle Salad with Fresh Vegetables

■

MAKES 4 SERVINGS

Fresh Asian noodles are sold in most supermarkets in the produce section with Asian vegetables.

3 tablespoons canola oil
1 teaspoon sesame oil
3 tablespoons rice vinegar
½ teaspoon sugar (omit if rice vinegar is seasoned)
¼ teaspoon salt (omit if rice vinegar is seasoned)
1 slice fresh ginger, finely minced
A few dashes of hot pepper sauce, such as Tabasco

6 ounces Asian-style noodles or American vermicelli
6 scallions, cut diagonally into 1-inch pieces
1 cup sliced radishes
1 large cucumber, seeded and cut into ½-inch slices
2 celery stalks, thinly sliced

Whisk together the canola oil, sesame oil, vinegar, sugar, salt, ginger, and hot pepper sauce to taste until the sugar and salt are dissolved.

In a large pot of rapidly boiling salted water, cook the noodles until tender but not mushy, about 1 minute for Asian noodles. For vermicelli, follow the package directions. Drain and rinse in cold water. In a large salad bowl, toss the noodles with the dressing. Add the vegetables and toss again. Serve at room temperature or chilled.

Kilocalories 247 Kc • Protein 5 gm • Fat 12 gm • Percent of calories from fat 43% • Cholesterol 3 mg • Dietary fiber 3 gm • Sodium 234 mg • Calcium 35 mg

Layered Nacho Salad

Choose a large glass bowl to show off the layers of this popular buffet salad.

1 (10-ounce) package
  frozen corn
1 medium head romaine lettuce,
  shredded
1 green bell pepper, seeded
  and diced
1 red bell pepper, seeded
  and diced
4 large carrots, coarsely grated
3 cups broken baked
  tortilla chips

3 cups homemade black beans
  (page 16) or 2 (14-ounce) cans
  low-sodium black beans,
  drained and rinsed
8 ounces grated Cheddar cheese
3 cups Guacamole (page 27)
3 cups Zesty Tomato Salsa (page
  18 or store-bought tomato
  salsa from a jar)

Cook the corn according to package directions; drain and cool.

Layer half the lettuce, bell peppers, carrots, corn, chips, beans, and cheese in a large salad bowl, preferably with straight sides. Add a layer of half the guacamole and half the salsa. Repeat with the remaining ingredients.

Kilocalories 388 Kc • Protein 19 gm • Fat 17 gm • Percent of calories from fat 37% • Cholesterol 20 mg • Dietary fiber 11 gm • Sodium 392 mg • Calcium 292 mg

SALADS

Green Vegetables Salad with Smoked Salmon

A crusty loaf of fresh rye bread is a great accompaniment to this luncheon salad.

½ pound fresh green beans
½ pound broccoli florets
1 green bell pepper, seeded and cut into strips
½ pound tender young spinach, washed, tough stems removed, and torn into bite-size pieces

1 tablespoon chopped fresh chives
About ½ cup Dijon Vinaigrette (page 20)
6 ounces sliced smoked salmon, cut into strips

Cook the green beans in boiling salted water until they are just tender, about 5 minutes. Remove them with a slotted spoon and rinse in cool water. Cook the broccoli florets in the same water until tender-crisp, 3 minutes. Drain and rinse in cool water.

Combine the vegetables in a large salad bowl. Blend the chives into ½ cup of the dressing. Toss the vegetables with the dressing, adding more if needed. Arrange the salmon in a fan on top and serve at once.

Kilocalories 288 Kc • Protein 13 gm • Fat 23 gm • Percent of calories from fat 68% • Cholesterol 10 mg • Dietary fiber 5 gm • Sodium 417 mg • Calcium 122 mg

ANTIOXIDANT POWER

344

Salad Niçoise

As you'll see when you read this ingredients list, almost anything savory or crunchy can be made part of this composed salad, so feel free to substitute what you have on hand. This provincial dish is a light meal in itself, needing only a long loaf of French bread for accompaniment.

1 red onion, peeled, sliced, and separated into rings

1 large head Bibb lettuce

1 cup fresh cooked green beans

2 medium ripe tomatoes, cut into wedges

1 large potato, cooked and sliced

4 to 6 raw cauliflower or broccoli florets, sliced

1 (7-ounce) can water-packed tuna, drained and flaked

2 hard-cooked eggs, peeled and sliced, or 1 cup cubed ricotta salata or feta cheese

½ cup pitted black olives, preferably brine-cured

About ½ cup Herb Vinaigrette (page 20) or Caesar Salad Dressing with Roasted Garlic (page 21)

Soak the onion rings in ice water for a half hour or so to sweeten them. Drain.

Layer the Bibb lettuce leaves on a platter. Arrange the green beans, tomatoes, potato, cauliflower or broccoli, tuna, egg or cheese, and olives in rows over the lettuce. Scatter the onion rings over the top. Cover and chill the salad.

Drizzle the salad with the dressing or pass it at the table.

Kilocalories 358 Kc • Protein 19 gm • Fat 23 gm • Percent of calories from fat 57% • Cholesterol 121 mg • Dietary fiber 4 gm • Sodium 449 mg • Calcium 69 mg

Desserts

———————◼———————

There's no need to think of desserts as something you must give up in order to be healthy. Instead, consider them to be another opportunity for investing your daily fare with even more antioxidants while giving yourself a delectable treat. A healthy homemade dessert that satisfies our "sweet tooth" also may prevent our succumbing to the temptations of candy bars and other empty calorie snacks.

The desserts in this chapter—such as Mango and Raspberry Compote, Oatmeal-Apricot Cake, and Pumpkin-Pecan Bread Pudding—are enriched with the fruits and vegetables that yield an abundance of vitamin C and beta-carotene and the grains, nuts, and oils that give us vitamin E. And they do make a gratifying conclusion to the main meal of the day.

Nonfat yogurt is a frequent ingredient in these low-fat desserts—in two forms. *Plain* nonfat yogurt is frequently used as an ingredient in "creamy" fruit dishes and in baked goods. *Frozen* nonfat yogurt is often suggested as a topping to replace the ice cream and whipped cream of yesteryear. Read each ingredient list carefully to know which is called for in that particular recipe.

Desserts that feature fresh antioxidant foods are easy to prepare and don't require a degree in the art of pastry making. They're also attractive, homestyle dishes you can be proud to serve to guests as well as family. So go ahead—indulge!

Shopping and Storing Savvy

Since fresh fruits are the basis of many antioxidant-rich desserts, you'll want to shop for these perishable items wisely and store them carefully. The following guide offers a few suggestions and tips to help you. As with vegetables, the best advice is to plan on using fruits seasonally—that is, make your strawberry creations in the spring and your apple desserts in the fall. You'll enjoy better fruits for less money if you stay with the seasonal specials.

Apples

Whenever possible, choose apples that haven't been waxed, since this coating prevents you from washing off any traces of dirt or pesticide that may be lurking underneath. The skins should be unblemished, the flesh unbruised and firm. Smaller apples may look like a better bargain, but they're liable to have a greater proportion of waste in seeds and core. Baldwin, Cortland, Granny Smith, Macoun, Rome, and Winesap are all good cooking apples. McIntosh, which cooks to a mush very easily, is great for sauce but not for cakes and tarts. Apples will keep at room temperature for a week or more, making them ideal for an attractive fruit bowl.

Apricots, Peaches, and Nectarines

Enjoy these summer beauties at the height of their season; out-of-season apricots, peaches, and nectarines hardly ever ripen properly. Look for plump, well-formed fruit with good characteristic color and scent. Slightly hard peaches and nectarines will soften if left at room temperature for a day or two; refrigerate them as soon as they are fully ripe. Unfortunately, a deplorable new supermarket trend is to paste code stickers on these delicate fruits. When you remove the stickers, a piece of skin often comes with them, so after washing the fruit, if the stickers don't slide off easily, leave them in place until ready to use the fruit.

Bananas

It's a bonus that bananas are available all year. Harvested green, they continue to ripen at room temperature. It's best to buy a bunch in which a few are still tinged with green, but if you do miscalculate and they all ripen too fast, refrigerate the extras. The skin will turn dark but you'll get two to three more days out of the fruit.

Berries

Look for bright fresh color and a sweet smell when buying berries. Stained cardboard containers may indicate that the bottom layer is crushed. Strawberries should retain their caps, but raspberries should not. Small wild blueberries have much more flavor than large cultivated ones and their size works better in baked goods as well. Refrigerate berries; when you're ready to use them, rinse them gently. Plan on using raspberries within one day, strawberries within three days. Blueberries may last up to five days.

Like other berries, cranberries have a short season, but you can freeze them. Later they can be chopped or poached without thawing. For this reason, it's wise to rinse and dry them well *before* freezing.

Citrus Fruits

Plentiful in winter, citrus fruits set the standard for vitamin C content. In the market, look for fruit that's firm but not hard, well rounded, and heavy for its size. A slightly greenish tinge on lemons and some varieties of oranges may be an indication of freshness rather than immaturity. It's worth your while to taste-test organically grown citrus fruits. They may be more expensive, but I find that they have that old-fashioned sweet flavor. Citrus fruits will keep a week or more in the refrigerator.

Mangoes and Papayas

Choose fruits that are unbruised and fragrant. Buy these two tropical treats when they are about half yellow, then finish ripening them at room temperature at home. They are ripe when the flesh yields slightly to pressure. If you're not ready to use them right then, refrigerate them for two to three more days.

Melons

Select melons that are unblemished, fragrant, and heavy. The hollow where the fruit was attached to the vine should be smooth, not jagged, indicating it was ready to slip off the vine when harvested. Refrigerate melons until ready to serve them.

The new seedless watermelons are a wonderful time-saver, encouraging you to eat more of this succulent antioxidant fruit. If you wish, you can peel, seed, and slice melons, then store them in a plastic container as an incentive for nutritious snacking.

Pears

Bosc pears are naturally firmer and keep their shape well when poached; D'Anjous are also good pears for cooking. Although Bartletts are terrific eating pears, their flesh when fully ripe is a bit soft for cooking. Since pears continue to ripen after picking, it's okay to buy really firm fruit and keep them at room temperature until they are soft and juicy. Like apples, pears are a fine choice for a fruit bowl arrangement.

Pineapple

Buy a pineapple that's firm and fragrant, with fresh-looking green leaves. A yellow skin does not necessarily indicate that a pineapple is ripe—a distinctive pineapple-y aroma is a better clue. Choose a larger size for less waste when you peel and core the fruit. Since a pineapple doesn't ripen any more once cut, it should be refrigerated after purchase.

Easiest Peaches Melba

The easy elegance of this colorful dessert makes it especially pleasing.

½ cup seedless raspberry or red
   currant jelly
1 cup fresh or frozen
   unsweetened raspberries
3 large fresh ripe peaches,
   peeled and sliced

3 tablespoons sugar
1 teaspoon vanilla extract
6 scoops frozen nonfat vanilla
   yogurt

In a small saucepan, melt the jelly and stir in the raspberries. If they are fresh, immediately remove from the heat. If frozen, bring the mixture to a simmer, then remove. Let the berries stand at room temperature for up to an hour. If kept longer, refrigerate, but bring to room temperature before using.

Toss the peach slices with the sugar. Sprinkle with the vanilla. Toss again and chill until needed.

When ready to serve, divide the peaches among 6 glass dessert dishes. Add a scoop of frozen yogurt. Top each with about ¼ cup sauce. Serve immediately.

Kilocalories 244 Kc • Protein 6 gm • Fat 0 gm • Percent of calories from fat 1% • Cholesterol 0 mg • Dietary fiber 3 gm • Sodium 96 mg • Calcium 122 mg

DESSERTS

351

Peach Melba Terrine

---■---

MAKES 6 SERVINGS

From the same tradition as the previous recipe, this is a beautiful molded version you'll be proud to serve.

4 large ripe peaches, peeled and
   sliced (see Note)
½ cup sugar
1 vanilla bean
2 packets unflavored gelatin
1 cup orange juice

1 (8-ounce) container nonfat
   peach, mango, apricot, or
   vanilla yogurt
1 cup fresh or frozen
   unsweetened raspberries

For the sauce

½ cup seedless raspberry or red
   currant jelly

¼ cup orange juice

In a medium saucepan, combine the peaches, ½ cup water, the sugar, and vanilla bean. Bring to a boil, stirring until the sugar is dissolved, and gently simmer the peaches until they are tender, 8 to 10 minutes. Remove the peaches with a slotted spoon. Remove and reserve the vanilla bean, which may be rinsed, dried, and used again.

Sprinkle the gelatin on the orange juice and let stand 5 minutes until softened. Stir the mixture into the poaching syrup and warm over low heat until the gelatin is dissolved. Cool slightly, then whisk in the yogurt.

Put the peaches into a nonstick loaf pan. Sprinkle the raspberries on top. Carefully pour in the gelatin mixture and chill the terrine, covered with plastic wrap, until set, 6 hours or overnight.

To make the sauce, melt the jelly over low heat and stir in the orange juice. Pour into a small pitcher and let stand, covered, until cooled to room temperature. If chilled, bring to room temperature before using.

Unmold the terrine by dipping it up to the rim in hot water; invert onto a platter. Pour 2 tablespoons berry sauce onto each dessert plate and top with a slice of the terrine.

NOTE: When fresh peaches are not in season, 1 (30-ounce) can peaches in light syrup can be substituted. Drain the peaches, reserving the liquid. Omit the water, sugar, and vanilla bean. Use 1 cup peach liquid in place of the poaching syrup, adding 1 teaspoon vanilla extract.

Kilocalories 234 Kc • Protein 3 gm • Fat 0 gm • Percent of calories from fat 1% • Cholesterol 0 mg • Dietary fiber 2 gm • Sodium 40 mg • Calcium 70 mg

Peaches and Strawberries with Grenadine

MAKES 4 SERVINGS

Grenadine is a nonalcoholic syrup made from pomegranates, usually for flavoring alcoholic drinks, available in liquor stores.

**2 large ripe peaches, peeled and
  sliced
1 pint strawberries, preferably
  large ones, hulled and sliced
⅓ cup grenadine syrup**

**4 mint sprigs for garnish
  (optional)
4 mint chocolate cookies
  (optional)**

Combine the peaches, strawberries, and grenadine. Chill to blend the flavors, stirring once or twice. Divide among 4 dessert dishes. To make the dessert a little more special, garnish with mint sprigs and serve with mint chocolate cookies.

Kilocalories 112 Kc • Protein 1 gm • Fat .33 gm • Percent of calories from fat 2% • Cholesterol 0 mg • Dietary fiber 3 gm • Sodium 13 mg • Calcium 14 mg

Individual Summer Puddings

MAKES 4 SERVINGS

This easy, lazy summer dessert that's a favorite in Britain deserves special notice for its outstanding nutritional value—lots of vitamin C!

4 cups raspberries and blueberries (any ratio)
½ cup sugar
4 slices firm white sandwich bread, crusts removed

Frozen nonfat vanilla yogurt as a topping (optional)

Combine the berries, sugar, and ⅓ cup water in a medium saucepan and bring to a boil, stirring often. Reduce the heat and simmer for 12 minutes, or until thick but pourable, stirring occasionally. Taste the sauce (carefully—it's hot!) to see if you want more sugar. If so, add up to 2 more tablespoons and cook until it's well dissolved. Cool the sauce slightly until it's just warm.

Select 4 goblets or large wineglasses and use one of them to cut rounds out of the bread slices. Save and chop the trimmings. Divide the trimmings among the wineglasses. Top each with ¼ cup sauce. Add the bread rounds and divide the remaining sauce among the glasses. Chill overnight. If desired, top with the frozen vanilla yogurt.

Kilocalories 215 Kc • Protein 3 gm • Fat 1 gm • Percent of calories from fat 5% • Cholesterol 0 mg • Dietary fiber 8 gm • Sodium 109 mg • Calcium 40 mg

Strawberries with Orange-Honey Yogurt

The easiest way to warm honey is to spoon it into a Pyrex cup and microwave it for a few seconds until the honey is liquid enough to mix with the other ingredients.

3 tablespoons honey, slightly warmed
1 teaspoon grated orange zest
1 cup nonfat plain yogurt

1 quart strawberries
6 teaspoons sugar
6 tablespoons orange juice

Whisk the honey and orange zest into the yogurt. Chill until needed.

Wash and hull the strawberries. Slice them into 6 dessert dishes. Sprinkle each portion with 1 teaspoon sugar and 1 tablespoon orange juice. Let them marinate for a half hour at room temperature or an hour in the refrigerator, stirring them once.

When ready to serve, top the strawberries with the yogurt.

Kilocalories 107 Kc • Protein 3 gm • Fat .40 gm • Percent of calories from fat 3% • Cholesterol 0 mg • Dietary fiber 2 gm • Sodium 30 mg • Calcium 92 mg

Mango and Raspberry Compote

Marinating dried fruits will plump and soften them as if they had been cooked.

1 ripe mango, peeled and diced
2 cups fresh or frozen
  unsweetened raspberries
10 dried apricots

¼ cup sugar
¼ cup orange juice
4 crisp chocolate cookies

Combine the mango and raspberries in a bowl. Snip the apricots into slices and add to the fruit. Stir the sugar into the orange juice and blend with the fruit. Chill at least 2 hours, stirring once or twice.

    Divide the fruit among 4 dessert dishes. Crush the cookies and sprinkle them on the fruit as a crunchy topping.

Kilocalories 217 Kc • Protein 2 gm • Fat 1 gm • Percent of calories from fat 5% • Cholesterol 0 mg • Dietary fiber 7 gm • Sodium 30 mg • Calcium 37 mg

ANTIOXIDANT POWER

356

Peach-Almond Sherbet

Don't substitute no-sugar-added canned fruit in this recipe. The texture of the sherbet depends on heavy syrup and there is no other sweetener in the dessert.

1 (16-ounce) can peaches in
   heavy syrup
¾ teaspoon natural almond
   flavoring

⅔ cup nonfat plain yogurt

The day before making the sherbet, empty the contents of the can of peaches into a plastic container and freeze it solidly.

Run warm water over the container to remove the block of peaches. Put the block in a pan or other sturdy container and break the block in half by piercing it in several places in a straight line on both sides; use a medium paring knife with a sharp point. Once this is done, place the 2 pieces on a breadboard and use a chef's knife to break it into chunks.

Transfer the chunks to a food processor and puree them. Blend in the flavoring and yogurt. Refreeze the sherbet. It's best used the same day but will still have a spoonable texture on the second day.

Kilocalories 109 Kc • Protein 3 gm • Fat .14 gm • Percent of calories from fat 1% • Cholesterol 0 mg • Dietary fiber 1 gm • Sodium 35 mg • Calcium 79 mg

APRICOT-LEMON SHERBET: Follow the preceding directions, substituting pitted apricot halves in heavy syrup for the peaches and ¼ teaspoon lemon extract for the almond flavoring.

Kilocalories 121 Kc • Protein 3 gm • Fat .15 gm • Percent of calories from fat 1% • Cholesterol 0 mg • Dietary fiber 2 gm • Sodium 41 mg • Calcium 86 mg

Summer Fruit Medley with Honey Yogurt

---

2 ripe peaches or nectarines,
   peeled and cut into bite-size
   chunks
1 pint fresh strawberries, hulled
   and quartered lengthwise
1 cup fresh raspberries
3 or more tablespoons honey,
   slightly warmed

½ teaspoon natural almond
   flavoring
1 cup nonfat plain yogurt
4 amaretti, crushed (Italian crisp
   almond cookies—optional)

Combine the fruits in a serving bowl. Whisk the honey and almond flavoring into the yogurt. Taste to check if you want more sweetener. Stir the yogurt into the fruit. Garnish with crushed amaretti, if desired; they add a delightful crunch. Serve immediately.

Kilocalories 280 Kc • Protein 8 gm • Fat 5 gm • Percent of calories from fat 18% • Cholesterol 0 mg • Dietary fiber 6 gm • Sodium 80 mg • Calcium 168 mg

ANTIOXIDANT POWER

Three-Berry Sundaes

These are for kids of all ages, as a dessert, or as an evening snack—packed with antioxidants and calcium as well.

1 pint fresh strawberries, hulled
  and quartered lengthwise
1 cup fresh raspberries
1 cup fresh blueberries
½ cup or more sugar
1 banana, peeled and cut
  lengthwise and crosswise—
  4 pieces

6 scoops frozen nonfat vanilla
  yogurt
6 crisp chocolate wafers
  (optional)

Combine the berries and sugar in a bowl and let them stand at room temperature until they begin to get juicy, stirring occasionally. Chill until needed. Stir before using and taste to see if the mixture is sweet enough for your taste.

To assemble the sundaes, divide the banana pieces among 4 glass dessert dishes. Add a spoonful of mixed berries to each. Add the frozen yogurt and top with the remaining berries. Garnish with the wafers, if desired.

Kilocalories 241 Kc • Protein 6 gm • Fat .48 gm • Percent of calories from fat 2% • Cholesterol 0 mg • Dietary fiber 3 gm • Sodium 89 mg • Calcium 128 mg

Baked Peaches and Blueberries
with Amaretti

■

This delectable dessert brings together antioxidant peaches and bacteria-fighting blueberries. These late-summer berries are high in anthocyanins, substances that help to fight infection.

2 large ripe peaches, peeled and
  sliced
1 cup fresh or frozen unthawed
  blueberries
2 tablespoons sugar

¼ teaspoon natural almond
  flavoring
4 amaretti cookies (Italian crisp
  almond cookies), crushed into
  crumbs

Preheat the oven to 350 degrees F.

Arrange the peaches in a buttered gratin dish or 8-inch pie pan. Scatter the blueberries over the top. Mix the sugar with the flavoring and sprinkle it over the fruit. Bake 20 to 25 minutes, until the peaches are tender, stirring once during the cooking time. Allow the fruit to cool until it's just warm. Divide it among 4 dessert dishes and top with the amaretti crumbs.

Kilocalories 205 Kc • Protein 4 gm • Fat 5 gm • Percent of calories from fat 24% • Cholesterol 0 mg • Dietary fiber 4 gm • Sodium 38 mg • Calcium 40 mg

ANTIOXIDANT POWER

360

Oranges in Lime-Mint Syrup

Cool and refreshing after a heavy dinner, this citrus dessert can be served as is or topped with a small scoop of lime sherbet.

½ cup dry vermouth or dry
  white wine
Juice of 1 lime (2 tablespoons)
4 strips of lime peel
⅓ cup sugar

2 tablespoons chopped
  fresh mint
3 large navel oranges, peeled, all
  pith removed, and sliced into
  ½-inch-thick rounds

Combine the wine, ½ cup water, lime juice, lime peel, and sugar in a saucepan. Bring to a boil, reduce the heat, and simmer the syrup for 8 minutes. Remove from the heat. Cool 5 minutes and stir in the mint.

Put the oranges in a glass bowl and pour the syrup over them. Chill at least 1 hour before serving.

Kilocalories 144 Kc • Protein 1 gm • Fat 0 gm • Percent of calories from fat 1% • Cholesterol 0 mg • Dietary fiber 3 gm • Sodium 3 mg • Calcium 50 mg

Baked Bananas and Apricots with Pecans

Apricots are a great source of beta-carotene, pecans provide the anti-oxidant mineral zinc, and bananas provide potassium and magnesium—two important heart protectors.

3 tablespoons unsalted butter, melted

3 bananas, peeled and cut into 1-inch pieces

12 dried apricots, cut in half

½ cup unsalted pecan halves or pieces

3 tablespoons brown sugar

¼ teaspoon ground nutmeg

Preheat the oven to 350 degrees F.

Put the melted butter into a medium gratin dish, add the fruit and nuts, and sprinkle with the sugar and nutmeg. Stir to coat all sides with the butter and sugar. Bake in the middle of the oven for 15 minutes, stirring once during the cooking time. Cool slightly and serve warm or at room temperature.

Kilocalories 304 Kc • Protein 3 gm • Fat 14 gm • Percent of calories from fat 39% • Cholesterol 11 mg • Dietary fiber 5 gm • Sodium 11 mg • Calcium 30 mg

Carrot Cup Custards

The carrots can be finely shredded or ground in a food processor. They will rise to the top of these custards and contribute a soft chewy layer, something like coconut.

1 tablespoon unsalted butter, melted

1 tablespoon plain dry bread crumbs

⅓ cup golden raisins

2 cups whole milk

2 eggs, beaten

⅓ cup sugar

¼ teaspoon plus more ground nutmeg

2 medium carrots, very finely shredded (1 cup, loosely packed)

Preheat the oven to 325 degrees F. Brush the insides of 6 heatproof custard cups with the melted butter. Coat the sides and bottoms with the bread crumbs. Set the cups in a baking dish. Soak the raisins in very hot water for 5 minutes; drain.

Beat together the milk, eggs, sugar, and ¼ teaspoon nutmeg until well blended. Stir in the raisins and carrots. Divide the mixture among the cups. Sprinkle a little more nutmeg on top of each. Set the pan holding the cups in the oven. Pour enough hot water into the outer pan to come halfway up the sides of the cups. Bake until golden and set, about 50 minutes. Cool on a rack before serving.

Kilocalories 170 Kc • Protein 5 gm • Fat 6 gm • Percent of calories from fat 28% • Cholesterol 84 mg • Dietary fiber 1 gm • Sodium 82 mg • Calcium 119 mg

Baked Papaya

———— ■ ————

After a heavy meat meal, this might be the perfect light dessert. A rich source of vitamin A, papaya also has enzymes that break down protein, making this tropical fruit a digestive aid as well.

3 firm, just-ripe papaya, peeled, seeded, and sliced

2 tablespoons unsalted butter, melted

2 tablespoons fresh lemon juice

3 tablespoons brown sugar

Ground cinnamon for sprinkling

Preheat the oven to 350 degrees F.

Put the papaya slices into a 13 × 9-inch glass or ceramic baking dish. Gently toss them with the melted butter and lemon juice, then arrange them in an attractive layer. Sprinkle with brown sugar and several dashes of cinnamon. Bake for 20 minutes, or until tender. Cool to warm before serving.

Kilocalories 98 Kc • Protein 1 gm • Fat 2 gm • Percent of calories from fat 19% • Cholesterol 5 mg • Dietary fiber 3 gm • Sodium 9 mg • Calcium 40 mg

BAKED MANGO: Follow the preceding recipe, substituting ripe mangoes for the papaya. Mangoes are tricky to peel and slice but worth the effort.

Kilocalories 111 Kc • Protein 1 gm • Fat 2 gm • Percent of calories from fat 17% • Cholesterol 5 mg • Dietary fiber 2 gm • Sodium 6 mg • Calcium 17 mg

Peach Cobbler with a Cornbread Topping

Whole grain cornmeal is sold in natural food stores; it's richer in vitamin E than refined cornmeal.

6 large ripe peaches, peeled and sliced

¼ cup brown sugar
¼ teaspoon ground cinnamon

Topping

1 cup unbleached all-purpose flour
½ cup cornmeal, preferably whole grain
¼ cup granulated sugar
1 teaspoon baking powder

½ teaspoon baking soda
1 large egg, beaten
½ cup nonfat plain yogurt
3 tablespoons vegetable oil
Additional ground cinnamon and sugar for sprinkling

Preheat the oven to 375 degrees F.

Put the peaches into a 9-inch glass pie pan or a 9-inch-square nonreactive baking dish. Mix them with the brown sugar and cinnamon.

Sift together the dry ingredients for the topping. Whisk together the egg, yogurt, and oil. Stir the liquid ingredients into the dry ingredients until just blended. Spoon the batter over the fruit and spread it to the edges of the pan. Sprinkle with a little cinnamon and sugar.

Bake in the top third of the oven for 20 to 25 minutes, until the top is golden brown and the peaches are tender. If the top browns too fast, lay a sheet of foil over it. Cool until just warm for serving.

Kilocalories 295 Kc • Protein 6 gm • Fat 8 gm • Percent of calories from fat 25% • Cholesterol 35 mg • Dietary fiber 3 gm • Sodium 204 mg • Calcium 86 mg

Pumpkin-Pecan Bread Pudding

MAKES 6 SERVINGS

Pumpkin for vitamin A and pecans and whole wheat for vitamin E make a dessert with antioxidant pizzazz.

3 large eggs
¾ cup mashed cooked pumpkin
   or canned unflavored pumpkin
   pie filling
⅔ cup brown sugar
½ teaspoon ground cinnamon
¼ teaspoon ground nutmeg

¼ teaspoon ground ginger
⅛ teaspoon ground cloves
⅛ teaspoon salt
1¼ cups low-fat milk
2 cups diced crustless whole
   wheat bread (about 3 slices)
½ cup pecan halves or pieces

Whip the eggs with a whisk until light. Beat in the pumpkin. Add the sugar, spices, and salt; blend well. Mix in the milk.

Put the bread into a 2½-quart glass casserole (preferably flat, 2 inches deep) set into a large baking pan. Pour the pumpkin mixture over all, pressing the bread down. Let stand for 15 minutes.

Preheat the oven to 350 degrees F.

Sprinkle the top of the pudding with the pecans. Place the baking dishes in the middle of the oven and pour hot water into the outer pan. Bake 40 to 45 minutes, until set at the center. Serve warm or at room temperature.

Kilocalories 250 Kc • Protein 7 gm • Fat 10 gm • Percent of calories from fat 35% • Cholesterol 110 mg • Dietary fiber 2 gm • Sodium 181 mg • Calcium 112 mg

Peach-Almond Crisp

■

As in many recipes, nectarines can be substituted for peaches with no other changes in the recipe. Being somewhat sweeter and denser, nectarines have a few more calories than peaches, but both fruits can be considered low-cal treats.

⅓ cup brown sugar
⅓ cup unbleached all-purpose flour
½ teaspoon natural almond flavoring
Pinch of salt
3 tablespoons unsalted butter

⅓ cup quick-cooking or old-fashioned uncooked oats
½ cup slivered blanched almonds
⅓ cup granulated sugar
6 ripe peaches or nectarines, peeled and sliced

Preheat the oven to 375 degrees F.

To make the topping, in a food processor, mix together the brown sugar, flour, ¼ teaspoon almond flavoring, and salt. Cut in the butter until the mixture is mealy. Add the oats and almonds. Process briefly until the almonds are coarsely chopped.

Alternatively, the almonds can be chopped by hand, the topping mixed in a bowl, and the butter cut in with a pastry cutter.

In a 10-inch glass pie pan, mix the granulated sugar, peaches, and remaining ¼ teaspoon almond flavoring. Press the fruit down into an even layer. Sprinkle the topping over all and press that into a layer.

Bake in the middle of the oven for 30 minutes, or until the fruit is tender and the topping is nicely browned. Serve warm from the pan.

Kilocalories 264 Kc • Protein 4 gm • Fat 11 gm • Percent of calories from fat 35% • Cholesterol 16 mg • Dietary fiber 3 gm • Sodium 66 mg • Calcium 50 mg

DESSERTS

Gingered Apple and Pear Crisp

MAKES 6 SERVINGS

A fruit crisp is a low-calorie, high-nutrition, and great-flavor alternative to pie!

⅓ cup granulated sugar

1 teaspoon ground ginger

3 large cooking apples, such as Granny Smith, Baldwin, Rome, or Macoun, peeled, cored, and thinly sliced

3 ripe Bosc or D'Anjou pears, peeled, cored, and thinly sliced

2 tablespoons finely chopped crystallized ginger (optional)

⅓ cup unbleached all-purpose flour

⅓ cup firmly packed brown sugar

⅛ teaspoon salt

3 tablespoons unsalted butter

½ cup quick-cooking or old-fashioned uncooked oats

Preheat the oven to 350 degrees F.

In a bowl, mix the granulated sugar with ½ teaspoon ground ginger, and toss with the apple and pear slices. Stir in the crystallized ginger, if using. Spoon the fruit into a flat baking dish, such as a 12-inch glass pie pan or gratin pan of similar size, and lightly press it into an even layer.

Mix together the flour, brown sugar, remaining ½ teaspoon ground ginger, and salt for the topping. Cut in the butter with a pastry cutter or 2 knives until the mixture is mealy. Blend in the oatmeal. Sprinkle the topping over the fruit. Bake for 35 minutes, or until the topping is golden and the fruit is tender. Serve warm or at room temperature.

Kilocalories 266 Kc • Protein 2 gm • Fat 4 gm • Percent of calories from fat 14% • Cholesterol 8 mg • Dietary fiber 5 gm • Sodium 56 mg • Calcium 24 mg

Oatmeal-Apricot Cake

This is an easy cake to make and bake for practically guiltless snacking.

1¼ cups boiling water
1 cup quick-cooking or old-
   fashioned uncooked oats
1½ cups unbleached all-
   purpose flour
1 teaspoon baking soda
1 teaspoon baking powder
½ teaspoon salt
¼ teaspoon ground cinnamon

¼ teaspoon ground allspice
¼ teaspoon ground ginger
¼ teaspoon ground nutmeg
1 cup dark brown sugar
2 eggs, beaten
⅓ cup vegetable oil
⅔ cup dried apricots, snipped
   into pieces with a kitchen
   scissors

Pour the boiling water over the oats and let them stand for a half hour or so.

Preheat the oven to 350 degrees F. Spray a 13 × 9-inch pan with cooking spray, or butter and flour it.

Sift together the flour, baking soda, baking powder, salt, and spices. With an electric mixer or by hand, beat together the oat mixture, brown sugar, eggs, and oil. Beat in the dry ingredients. Fold in the apricots. Spoon the batter into the prepared pan.

Bake in the middle of the oven until a cake tester inserted in the center comes out dry, about 25 minutes. Cool in the pan on a wire rack.

Kilocalories 230 Kc • Protein 4 gm • Fat 8 gm • Percent of calories from fat 29% • Cholesterol 35 mg • Dietary fiber 2 gm • Sodium 255 mg • Calcium 40 mg

Peach Gingerbread

Powdered buttermilk is a convenient way to have this useful ingredient on hand whenever needed. To substitute powdered buttermilk for fresh, follow the instructions on the container.

1 (15- to 16-ounce) can peaches, no sugar added, well drained
1⅔ cups unbleached all-purpose flour
½ teaspoon baking soda
¼ teaspoon salt
1 large egg

½ cup dark molasses
⅓ cup vegetable oil
½ cup sugar
1 teaspoon ground ginger
1 teaspoon ground cinnamon
½ cup buttermilk

Preheat the oven to 350 degrees F. Spray a 9-inch-square pan with cooking spray. Dice the peaches and continue to drain them in a strainer until you're ready to add them to the batter. It's important that they be as dry as possible.

Sift together the flour, soda, and salt. In a large bowl, beat together the egg, molasses, oil, sugar, and spices until well blended. Add the flour mixture and buttermilk alternately in several portions, beginning and ending with flour and beating well after each addition. Fold in the peaches and turn the batter into the prepared pan.

Bake in the middle of the oven for 30 to 35 minutes, or until a cake tester inserted in the center comes out dry. Cool in the pan on a rack.

Kilocalories 257 Kc • Protein 4 gm • Fat 9 gm • Percent of calories from fat 30% • Cholesterol 24 mg • Dietary fiber 1 gm • Sodium 175 mg • Calcium 151 mg

Apricot-Chocolate Cheesecake

Make the yogurt cheese several hours or the night before preparing this recipe. It's a really low-fat cheesecake, with a topping of beta-carotene–rich apricots—so go ahead and indulge!

2 cups nonfat plain yogurt
6 small vanilla cookies or 3
  medium shortbread cookies
½ teaspoon unsalted butter
1 cup skim-milk ricotta cheese
¼ cup unsweetened cocoa
⅔ cup sugar
2 tablespoons cornstarch
1 large whole egg

1 egg white
1 teaspoon vanilla extract
½ teaspoon grated lemon zest
½ cup apricot preserves or
  apple jelly
1 (16-ounce) can apricot halves
  in juice pack, well drained and
  cut in half

Set a paper coffee filter in a strainer that will hold 2 cups, spoon the yogurt into it, and set it over a bowl. Cover with plastic wrap. Allow the yogurt to drain several hours or overnight in the refrigerator. Remove the thickened yogurt to a bowl and discard the liquid. You should have 1 cup yogurt cheese.

In a food processor, process the cookies until they are reduced to about ½ cup crumbs. Butter an 8-inch glass cake pan or 9-inch glass pie pan, and sprinkle the bottom and sides of the pan with the crumbs. Chill the pan.

Preheat the oven to 325 degrees F.

Beat together the yogurt, ricotta, cocoa, sugar, cornstarch, whole egg, egg white, and flavoring extracts until well blended. Slowly and gently pour the mixture into the prepared pan so as not to disturb the crumbs, and bake in the middle of the oven for 40 to 45 minutes, or until a table knife inserted near the center comes out clean. Cool completely.

Melt the jelly in a small saucepan. Arrange the apricots, rounded sides up, in a circle on the cheesecake. Use a pastry brush to paint the fruit with the melted jelly. Chill the cake again to set the jelly before serving.

Kilocalories 339 Kc • Protein 12 gm • Fat 7 gm • Percent of calories from fat 17% • Cholesterol 49 mg • Dietary fiber 2 gm • Sodium 170 mg • Calcium 295 mg

DESSERTS

Double Apple Spice Cake

This is a moist rich cake that's very low in fat while doubling up on apples. Walnuts are a good source of vitamin E.

2½ cups unbleached
  all-purpose flour
1 cup granulated sugar
1 teaspoon ground cinnamon
1 teaspoon ground ginger
½ teaspoon ground allspice
½ teaspoon ground nutmeg
2 teaspoons baking soda
1 teaspoon baking powder
½ teaspoon salt
¼ cup dark brown sugar

2 eggs
1 cup nonfat plain yogurt
1 cup applesauce
⅓ cup vegetable oil
1 cup peeled, finely diced apple,
  such as Cortland or Rome
⅔ cup plumped raisins (see
  Note, page 269)
⅔ cup coarsely chopped
  unsalted walnuts

Preheat the oven to 350 degrees F. Butter and flour a tube cake pan with a removable rim.

Sift together the flour, granulated sugar, cinnamon, ginger, allspice, nutmeg, baking soda, baking powder, and salt. Blend in the brown sugar.

Whisk together the eggs, yogurt, applesauce, and oil. Stir the liquid ingredients into the dry ingredients and beat to blend well. Fold in the diced apple, raisins, and walnuts. Spoon the batter into the prepared pan and level the top with a spatula.

Bake the cake in the middle of the oven for about 45 minutes, until it shrinks away slightly from the sides of the pan and is dry inside when tested with a cake tester. Cool the cake in the pan on a wire rack for 5 minutes. Remove the outer rim of the pan. When the cake has cooled enough to handle the remainder of the pan comfortably, remove it from the rest of the pan. Cool completely on a wire rack.

Kilocalories 328 Kc • Protein 7 gm • Fat 11 gm • Percent of calories from fat 30% • Cholesterol 35 mg • Dietary fiber 2 gm • Sodium 369 mg • Calcium 75 mg

Hidden Treasures Chocolate Cake

■

Here's a chocolate cake with a delicious crunch that you can feel good about, since its "hidden treasures" are beta-carotene–rich pumpkin plus vitamin E in the walnuts and Grape-Nuts (a wheat and barley cereal).

1 cup unbleached all-purpose flour	1 cup sugar
½ cup unsweetened cocoa	½ cup vegetable oil
1 teaspoon baking powder	1 cup mashed cooked pumpkin or canned unflavored pumpkin pie filling
½ teaspoon baking soda	
¼ teaspoon salt	
½ teaspoon ground cinnamon	½ cup finely chopped unsalted walnuts
¼ teaspoon ground ginger	½ cup Grape-Nuts cereal, not flakes (optional, or substitute another ½ cup walnuts)
¼ teaspoon ground allspice	
2 large eggs	

Preheat the oven to 350 degrees F. Spray a 9-inch-square pan with cooking spray, line it with wax paper, and spray the paper, too.

Sift together the flour, cocoa, baking powder, baking soda, salt, and spices. In the large bowl of an electric mixer, beat the eggs until they are light. Beat in the sugar, then the oil, then the pumpkin. Add the dry ingredients and beat until well blended. Fold in the walnuts and Grape-Nuts.

Spoon the batter into the prepared pan and bake in the middle of the oven for 35 to 40 minutes, or until a cake tester inserted in the center comes out dry. Cool the cake for 10 minutes in the pan on a rack. Loosen the sides with a table knife, invert onto another rack, and strip off the paper. Turn the cake upright and cool completely.

Kilocalories 350 Kc • Protein 6 gm • Fat 19 gm • Percent of calories from fat 49% • Cholesterol 53 mg • Dietary fiber 1 gm • Sodium 227 mg • Calcium 58 mg

DESSERTS

Putting It All Together—
Antioxidant-Rich Menus

For everydays and special days, you can use the recipes in this book to plan menus featuring the wonderful antioxidant foods in powerful, satisfying, and delicious combinations. More than just serving the occasional healthful dish, why not make antioxidant-rich foods the basis of a new style of dining—one that will defend you against the damage of free radicals. Stay healthier and younger by stressing the important antioxidant vitamins and minerals in your food choices all year long.

The menus in this section are designed to illustrate some pleasing possibilities. The number of servings is adjusted to the main course; in some cases you may have a little salad or dessert left over. You can, of course, mix and match recipes in a menu, substituting one dish for another, according to your individual taste and the preparation time available. The important thing is to enjoy the antioxidant foods in healthful, seasonal abundance.

A Light Spring Luncheon for Six

Chilled Red Bell Pepper Soup with Basil (*page 64*)
Asparagus and Vermicelli Frittata (*page 156*)
Whole Grain Italian Bread
Strawberries with Orange-Honey Yogurt (*page 355*)

An Outdoor-Indoor Dinner for Four

Southwestern Corn, Bean, and Cabbage Salad (*page 322*)
Grilled Tuna Kebabs with Vegetables (*page 144*)
Hot Brown Rice
Peach Cobbler with a Cornbread Topping (*page 365*) or Fresh Peaches

A Starlit Summer Supper for Four

Carrot Vichyssoise (*page 54*)
Broiled Swordfish with Warm Tomato Salad (*page 138*)
Broccoli with Walnut Dressing (*page 302*)
Whole grain French Bread
Watermelon Wedges

A July Dinner for Four

Baba Ghanouj with Roasted Garlic (*page 30*)
Whole Wheat Pita Bread
Poached Salmon with New Potatoes and Peas (*page 146*)
Tossed Greens with Tomato and Cucumber (*page 291*)

A Picnic for Six

Sliced Chicken Breast (*page 10*) Sandwiches on Light Rye Bread
Zucchini and Red Bell Pepper Frittata (*page 157*)
Potato and Broccoli Salad with Dijon Dressing (*page 330*)
Picnic Coleslaw (*page 317*)
Cantaloupe Wedges and Molasses Cookies

A Mostly Make-ahead Summer Dinner for Four

Chicken and Mixed Vegetable Salad (*page 127*)
Whole Wheat Pita Bread
Corn on the Cob
Bell Pepper Medley with Fresh Herbs (*page 229*)
Individual Summer Puddings (*page 354*) or Fresh Apricots

An Easy After-work Supper for Four

Tofu and Broccoli with Shells (*page 92*)
Carrot Slaw with Scallions (*page 319*)
Sesame Seed Bread or Rolls
Fresh Ripe Pears with a Bowl of Nuts

A Robust Fall Farmhouse Dinner for Four

Pork Chops Normandy with Cabbage and Sweet Potatoes (*page 135*)
Bell Pepper Corn Bread (*page 273*)
Peach-Almond Crisp (*page 367*)

A Vegetarian Feast for Four

Butternut and Bell Pepper Chowder (*page 66*)
Cabbage Rolls with Pistachio Brown-and-Wild Rice (*page 166*)
Navy Bean Salad with Scallions (*page 312*)
Crusty Rye Bread
Fresh Mango Slices

An Asian Dinner for Four

Subgum Vegetables with Tofu (*page 162*)
Chinese Green Bean Salad (*page 307*)
Hot Brown Rice
Fresh Pineapple Slices with Mint Sprigs

A Tea Party for Eight

Spiced Carrot Brown Bread (*page 272*)
Sweet Butter and a Selection of Preserves
Pineapple-Pear Muffins (*page 282*)
Double Apple Spice Cake (*page 372*)
Hot Tea, Milk, Sliced Lemon

A Hearty Luncheon for Four

Riso con Piselli (Italian Rice and Peas Soup) (*page 63*)
A Platter of Boiled Shrimp (*page 18*) with Garlic and Lemon Vinaigrette
(*page 19*)
Bruschetta with Tomato and Provolone (*page 40*)
Pineapple Sherbet with Mint Sprigs

An October Dinner Party for Four

Halloween Pumpkin and Apple Soup (*page 69*)
Chicken Breasts with Braised Cabbage (*page 120*)
Walnut 'n Wheat-stuffed Mushrooms (*page 38*)
Oatmeal-Apricot Cake (*page 369*)

An Informal Dinner for Six

Turkey Loaf with Shell Beans (*page 131*)
Colcannon with Kale and Leeks (*page 221*)
Carrot Slaw with Pineapple and Raisins (*page 320*)
Sliced Apples with Honey and Walnuts

A Holiday Dinner for Four

Crudités with Herb Aioli (*page 26*)
Roast Chicken
Mashed Potatoes with Caramelized Onions (*page 242*)
Baked Butternut Squash with Maple-Walnut Apples (*page 251*)
Brussels Sprouts with Dill and Celery Seed (*page 201*)
Tossed Greens with Fennel (*page 291*)
Mango and Raspberry Compote (*page 356*)

A Comforting Winter Supper for Four

All-Vegetable Shepherd's Pie (*page 173*)
Easy Whole Wheat Dinner Rolls (*page 268* or bakery-bought)
Oranges in Lime-Mint Syrup (*page 361*) or Tangerines

A Savory Brunch for Four

Grapefruit Juice
Baked Papaya (*page 364*)
Huevos Rancheros (*page 158*)
Whole Wheat Toast Triangles
Polenta Pronto (*page 12*)
Coffee

An Appetizer Buffet for Eight

Curry and Onion Cheese with Shrimp and Vegetables (*page 25*)
Hummus (*page 28*) with Whole Wheat Pita Bread
Sicilian Eggplant Caponata (*page 32*) with French Bread
Crabmeat-stuffed Cherry Tomatoes (*page 36*)
Marinated Cauliflower (*page 34*)
Layered Nacho Salad (*page 343*) with Baked Tortilla Chips

Index

INDEX